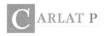

PRESCRIBING PSYCHOTROPICS

From Drug Interactions to Pharmacogenetics

FOURTH EDITION

(Previously *Drug Metabolism in Psychiatry*)

Chris Aiken, MD

Editor-in-chief of *The Carlat Psychiatry Report*, host of *The Carlat Psychiatry Podcast*, and director of the Mood Treatment Center in North Carolina

Joshua D. Feder, MD

Editor-in-chief of *The Carlat Child Psychiatry Report*, contributor to *The Carlat Psychiatry Podcast*, practicing psychiatrist in Solana Beach, CA, and medical director at Positive Development

Daniel J. Carlat, MD

Publisher of *The Carlat Psychiatry Report*, *The Carlat Child Psychiatry Report*, *The Carlat Addiction Treatment Report*, and *The Carlat Hospital Psychiatry Report*, and associate clinical professor at Tufts University School of Medicine, Boston, MA

Published by Carlat Publishing, LLC
PO Box 626, Newburyport, MA 01950
Copyright © 2022 All Rights Reserved.

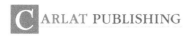
CARLAT PUBLISHING

Prescribing Psychotropics: From Drug Interactions to Pharmacogenetics
FOURTH EDITION
(Previously *Drug Metabolism in Psychiatry*)

Published by Carlat Publishing, LLC
PO Box 626, Newburyport, MA 01950

Publisher and Editor-in-Chief: Daniel J. Carlat, MD
Deputy Editor: Talia Puzantian, PharmD, BCPP
Executive Editor: Janice Jutras

This CME/CE activity is intended for psychiatrists, psychiatric nurses, psychologists, and other health care professionals with an interest in mental health. The Carlat CME Institute is accredited by the Accreditation Council for Continuing Medical Education to provide continuing medical education for physicians. Carlat CME Institute maintains responsibility for this program and its content. Carlat CME Institute designates this enduring material educational activity for a maximum of ten (10) AMA PRA Category 1 Credits™. Physicians or psychologists should claim credit commensurate only with the extent of their participation in the activity. The American Board of Psychiatry and Neurology has reviewed *Prescribing Psychotropics: From Drug Interactions to Pharmacogenetics* and has approved this program as part of a comprehensive Self-Assessment and CME Program, which is mandated by ABMS as a necessary component of maintenance of certification. CME tests must be taken online at www.thecarlatreport.com or https://www.thecarlat report.com/about/about-cme-center (for ABPN SA course subscribers).

To order, visit www.thecarlatreport.com or call (866) 348-9279

1 2 3 4 5 6 7 8 9 10

ISBN: 978-1-7329522-6-3
eISBN: 978-1-7329522-7-0

PRINTED IN THE UNITED STATES OF AMERICA

Table of Contents

Acknowledgments

For invaluable assistance, the authors wish to acknowledge:

Paul Carlat, MD, a wonderful father and psychiatrist, who test drove the book in his own practice.

Cal Colarusso, MD, a mentor who offers a full appreciation of the developmental lifespan.

Bernard Lee, MD, whose clinical judgement is a foundation for rational care of patients.

Charley Mitchell, of Lippincott Williams & Wilkins, for mentoring and teaching in the ways of publishing.

Richard Naimark, MD, a great psychiatrist, brother-in-law, and possessor of incredible common sense.

Xavier Preud'homme, MD, whose insatiable curiosity inspires the same in others.

Talia Puzantian, PharmD, BCPP, whose wealth of knowledge and wise guidance are a pillar of all of our publications at Carlat.

Sarah Rivelli, MD, for bringing judgement to uncertainty.

Neil Sandson, MD, for generosity of advice and encouragement.

Richard Weisler, MD, whose breadth of knowledge is matched only by his humility.

Marcia Zuckerman, MD, an editorial board member of *The Carlat Psychiatry Report* and quite possibly the most talented person on earth at making medical prose both relevant and comprehensible.

The members of the editorial boards of our four newsletters, who provide guidance and (most importantly) read and vet articles month after month after month.

Our outstanding Carlat staff, particularly our editorial team of Janice Jutras and Ilana Fogelson, who keep us pointed in the right direction.

And our patients and their families, whose experiences and questions give us the impetus to learn more and provide better care.

Preface

Most of our education as psychiatrists consists of learning how to diagnose patients and then learning how to choose the right treatment. This is important stuff. For example, I recently admitted a 36-year-old woman to the inpatient unit. The day before, she had been observed by neighbors trying to open the doors of several other apartments in her complex. When confronted, she screamed at them and said that "all these domiciles are my own." The police were called, and she was admitted on an involuntary basis to our unit.

My training enabled me to quickly establish rapport, arrive at a diagnostic differential (I entertained bipolar disorder, schizophrenia, and schizoaffective disorder, among others), and efficiently ask the right questions to rule those diagnoses in or out. I decided that she was suffering a manic episode, and my psychopharmacology training directed me to the most efficacious cocktail for quelling acute mania—a combination of a mood stabilizer, an antipsychotic, and a benzodiazepine.

But here's where the difficult decisions really begin, for this patient and others like her. Which mood stabilizer? I chose lithium. But which version of lithium? Should I start it in the morning or at night? How frequently should I dose it? When should I draw a blood level? Should I worry about other drugs the patient might be taking, such as ibuprofen for a sprained ankle?

The secret of excellent psychiatric treatment lies in the detailed answers to such questions. Over the course of our careers, we gradually learn about how different formulations of a given drug can make a big difference, how timing blood draws helps us titrate doses, how drugs can interact with one another, etc. But these lessons take many years to learn, and the answers change periodically as we learn more and with the development of new medications, new kinds of medications, and new technologies such as pharmacogenetics. There are few textbooks that focus explicitly on the details of drug metabolism and formulation—details that end up making the difference between superior treatment and treatment that is just "good enough."

That's why I wrote the first edition of this book, back in 2005. I fancifully titled it *When Molecules Collide*, not realizing that prospective readers would mistake it for a science fiction book. The second and third editions were retitled *Drug Metabolism in Psychiatry*—very faithful to the contents, but a title to go to sleep by. For the fourth edition, I teamed up with my colleagues Chris Aiken and Josh Feder to produce an expanded book, and decided to give it the somewhat more titillating title *Prescribing Psychotropics: From Drug Interactions to Pharmacogenetics.*

I hope you like it.

Daniel J. Carlat, MD
Newburyport, MA
November, 2021

SECTION I

The Basics

CHAPTER 1

Introduction: An Overview of Drug Metabolism and a Road Map to the Book

LET'S BEGIN THIS JOURNEY with a very basic question. Why do we need drug metabolism at all?

The best thinking among pharmacologists is that metabolism started when early organisms realized that they could improve their chances of survival by producing toxins and delivering them to potential predators. While poisoning enemies was good fun, a problem arose: how to avoid poisoning themselves. Metabolic enzyme systems therefore initially evolved in order to get rid of these endogenous toxins, but they turned out to be quite good at neutralizing exogenous toxins as well, such as food byproducts and (fast-forward a billion years) modern pharmaceuticals.

In order for drugs to work, they need to get into our system and into our cells. First, that means that the drug molecules have to be packaged in a delivery system that patients find attractive and are willing to swallow (see Chapter 2 on the secrets of pills and capsules)—or, sometimes they might be more efficiently delivered as patches, intranasally, or as injectables (see Chapters 6 and 7). Once the medications get into our system, they have to be absorbed and distributed. For GI absorption to happen, the stomach must grind down pills and capsules so that the molecules can come into contact with intestinal villi, where most of the actual absorption into the bloodstream takes place.

To effectively prescribe drugs, you need to know a bit about pharmacokinetics, which is the study of how long drugs stick around inside the body and what concentrations they typically achieve. The most clinically relevant parameters are half-life and area under the curve (AUC). The half-life is a measure of how rapidly half the amount of a drug is excreted, and the AUC represents the entire amount of drug that is present in the blood over a given period of time. Chapter 4 focuses on half-life, steady state, and the whole field of pharmacokinetics.

After drugs have worked their magic, we have to get rid of them. How do we accomplish this? The answer, which we discuss in Chapters 8 and 9, is that we transform them into water-soluble versions of themselves, so that they can be swept away in (watery) urine or stool. To do this, we use cytochrome P450 enzymes and glucuronidation, which you'll learn about in Chapter 8 as well.

By the way, as part of our effort to explain drug excretion in Chapter 9, we offer you our take on the kidney, that intimidating organ that we all know we should know more about but have been studiously avoiding. We show you that the kidney is made up of nephrons that do the work of drug excretion, and how understanding the process of tubule absorption will help you feel comfortable prescribing lithium and knowing when to order lithium levels.

Before drugs get excreted, they spend some time in the bloodstream, hopefully getting into the brain and doing something constructive for our patients (see Chapter 3 for an explanation of the blood-brain barrier). Along the way, they may encounter other drugs, leading to drug-drug interactions. We cover such interactions in Chapters 10, 11, and 12, and also focus on drug-food interactions that aren't as well known (Chapter 13) and interactions with recreational drugs (Chapter 14).

In Chapter 15 we cover the very important topic of *pharmacodynamic* interactions, in which some of our drugs combine forces with other drugs to cause potentially fatal assaults on the brain, such as serotonin syndrome and MAOI-induced hypertension. In that same chapter, we remind you of the dangers of anticholinergic interactions and how to minimize them in your patients.

Throughout the text, we try to keep a practical eye on how these concepts apply to your prescription pad. Toward that end, the new edition features more extensive coverage of three trends that have expanded since the first edition came out in 2005. More drugs have gone generic (Chapter 16), and a dizzying array of new formulations have become available, from delayed-release mechanisms to fast-acting dissolvable tablets (Chapters 5–7).

The third area of growth is pharmacogenetic testing, which we cover in Chapter 17. We explain the ever-controversial field of CYP450 genotyping and discuss whether commercial genetic panels are ever worth ordering. The final chapters (18–20) remind us of patient characteristics that can alter drug metabolism but do not require a genetic test to detect: age, gender, and ethnicity.

Don't forget the appendix, which brings the most useful charts and tables together for easy reference.

CHAPTER 2

Pills, Capsules, and Wafers: How Drugs Are Formulated and Why It Matters

A PSYCHOPHARMACOLOGIST PRESCRIBES thousands of pills over a career but is likely to have very little idea of how those medications are manufactured and formulated. In this chapter, we'll help to remedy this knowledge gap.

Some Definitions

The word "pill" comes from the Latin *pillula*, meaning a little ball or pellet. The term was first used in its medical sense in the 1400s and referred to a package of medicinal herbs with inert substances rolled into a sphere.

In modern usage, "pill" and "tablet" are interchangeable and refer to solid forms of medicines. They are manufactured by combining the powderized active molecule with inactive fillers called *excipients*. Those ingredients are then compressed together into a shape and size that is easily swallowed. The excipients are used for various reasons, including to bulk up the medicine so it's big enough to handle; to give the outer layer a pleasing taste, texture, or color; to help preserve the medicine; and to enhance the medicine's ability to effectively dissolve in the GI tract.

Unlike pills and tablets, capsules are not solid. Capsules are dissolvable shells that contain a powder or liquid form of the medication.

VEGAN MEDICINES?

Many capsule shells are made of gelatin from animal collagen, but recently there's been a shift toward plant derivatives. Unfortunately for your vegan or vegetarian patients, it is very difficult to determine if a given medication contains animal products. One study in Britain looked at the ingredients of the 100 most commonly prescribed medications in the National Health Service. Two-thirds of them contained ingredients that were potentially of animal origin, but the researchers were unable to determine that with greater precision. At this point, if you have a vegan patient who asks you about this issue, you should counsel them to reach out to the manufacturer directly.

Pills vs Capsules

Pills and tablets have a few advantages over capsules: lower cost, ease of cutting them in half, and longer shelf life. Their disadvantages include that they are typically harder to swallow and can have a bitter taste.

Liquid formulations are another common option to try when people have trouble swallowing medications. Many classes of psychotropic medications, including antipsychotics, antidepressants, stimulants, and anticonvulsants, are available in liquid form, and many more can be turned into a liquid by a compounding pharmacy. Liquids are also useful when patients have to taper off a medication very slowly to prevent withdrawal effects.

TABLE 2-1. Pros and Cons of Pills and Capsules

Pills and Tablets	Capsules
Harder to swallow but usually can be crushed (as long as they aren't extended or delayed release)	Easier to swallow
Can have bitter taste	Tasteless, odorless
Most can be cut in half	Most can be opened and mixed into foods or liquids
Longer shelf life, often lower cost	The power of suggestion: Capsules enhance the placebo response

TABLE 2-2. Prescription Abbreviations, Decoded

Abbreviation	Latin Term	Meaning
Rx	Recipe	Prescription
QD	Quaque die	Once a day
BID	Bis in die	Twice a day
TID	Ter in die	Three times a day
QID	Quater in die	Four times a day
HS	Hora somni	At bedtime
Q4h	Quaque 4 hora	Every four hours
PO	Per os	By mouth

Tough Pills to Swallow

Difficulty swallowing is a common cause of non-adherence, but it can also be dangerous. A pill that gets stuck going down can cause esophagitis and delayed absorption. This is why we advise patients to take their medication with a glass of water or with applesauce, yogurt, or a thick liquid. Patients with dysphagia should avoid thin liquids, which can cause aspiration.

Patients young and old can get creative with this. We've heard of success with ingesting meds mixed with peanut butter, whipped cream, M&Ms, or cake decorating sprinkles. Special devices are available to make swallowing easier, but most lack evidence. The do-it-yourself methods below were tested in a study of 151 adults and improved their ability to swallow medications 60%–89% of the time (Schiele JT et al, *Ann Fam Med* 2014;12(6):550–552).

Water Bottle Method for Tablets

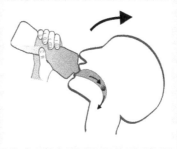

1. Fill a flexible plastic water bottle (the kind you could crush by sucking on the opening) with water.
2. Place the tablet on your tongue and close your lips tightly around the bottle. Then drink the water by sucking it down. Your lips should form a tight seal to keep air from getting in the bottle, so that the bottle squeezes in on itself as you suck the water down. Don't let air get into the bottle.

Lean-Forward Method for Capsules

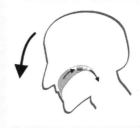

1. Place the capsule on your tongue.
2. Take a medium sip of water, but don't swallow yet.
3. Bend your head down by tilting your chin toward your chest and swallow the water and capsule.

TABLE 2-3. Techniques to Improve Swallowing

Swallowing Aid	Success Rate
Pill-swallowing cups	Unstudied (eg, Oralflo)
Pill-swallowing straws	Unstudied (eg, SafeStraw)
Pill-coating devices	Medcoat improved swallowing and taste in 98%–99%
Lubricant gels	Unstudied
Lubricant sprays	Pill Glide improved swallowing in 60%
Water bottle method for tablets	Improved swallowing in 60%
Lean-forward method for capsules	Improved swallowing in 89%

Orally Disintegrating Formulations

Orally disintegrating tablets (ODTs) have come on the scene over the last 20 years. Two of the most popular are olanzapine and mirtazapine ODT (formerly branded as Zyprexa Zydis and Remeron SolTab), but there are many others (see chart on page 11). In this section, we'll discuss some of the potential advantages of ODTs and describe various situations in which you might consider prescribing them.

ODTs are designed to dissolve quickly on the tongue. The first ODTs were vitamins that fizzed up in order to make them more pleasant for children. To achieve this, pharmaceutical companies used "loose-compression tableting," which is just as it sounds: a process where the tablets are compressed under low force. Loosely compressed tablets take about 20 seconds to dissolve. The FDA says that in order to be called an ODT, a tablet has to dissolve within 30 seconds.

An advance on the loose-compression technology is the Zydis technology, which was developed in the 1990s by R.P. Scherer Corporation. This process involves freeze-drying the various ingredients, resulting in pills that dissolve within 3 seconds. The first FDA-approved ODT was a Zydis form of Claritin in 1996. Klonopin Zydis ("wafers") was approved in 1997, and Zyprexa Zydis was approved in 2000.

ODT formulations are especially helpful for the following types of patients:

- Patients who don't like to swallow pills. According to some figures, this includes up to 35% of the general population and is especially common in psychiatric patients, children, and elderly patients.

- Patients with dysphagia (difficulty swallowing). This is especially common among elderly patients in nursing homes, where up to 60% have dysphagia.
- Disabled or bedridden patients who may not have easy access to water.
- Noncompliant patients who fake swallowing pills by cheeking them.

Another potential advantage of ODTs is that they may have a faster onset of action because some of the dissolved medication gets absorbed directly into the oral mucosa, avoiding the delays of the first-pass effect.

ODTs have at least two disadvantages. They are more expensive than regular pills, even after they've gone generic, and most of them can't be cut (some can, but the patient has to throw the remaining half of the pill away). Most of the ODTs in Table 2-4 have lost their patent, with the exception of two stimulants—Adzenys and Cotempla—that are slated for generic release in 2026.

TABLE 2-4. Orally Disintegrating Psychotropics

Generic Name	Orally Disintegrating Version
Aripiprazole	Aripiprazole ODT (Abilify Discmelt)
Asenapine	Asenapine sublingual (Saphris)
Clozapine	Clozapine ODT (FazaClo)
Olanzapine	Olanzapine ODT (Zyprexa Zydis)
Risperidone	Risperidone ODT (Risperdal M-Tab)
Mirtazapine	Mirtazapine ODT (Remeron SolTab)
Lamotrigine	Lamotrigine ODT
Amphetamine salts	Adzenys XR ODT
Methylphenidate	Cotempla XR ODT
Alprazolam	Alprazolam ODT (Niravam)
Clonazepam	Clonazepam ODT (Klonopin Wafers)
Zolpidem	Zolpidem sublingual (Edluar, Intermezzo) Zolpidem oral spray (Zolpimist)
Diphenhydramine	Diphenhydramine ODT (Benadryl FastMelt, Unisom SleepMelts)
Buprenorphine/ naloxone	Buprenorphine/naloxone sublingual tablet or film (Suboxone)
Donepezil	Donepezil ODT

A Closer Look at Olanzapine ODT

Olanzapine ODT (Zyprexa Zydis) has achieved something of a niche in the treatment of agitated and psychotic patients in emergency rooms and inpatient settings. While many such patients require restraints and involuntary intramuscular medication cocktails such as haloperidol/lorazepam/diphenhydramine, others are willing to take oral meds. For these patients, we need medications that get into the system as quickly and reliably as possible, which brings us to the orally disintegrating antipsychotic.

In an effort to determine if the ODT form of olanzapine has advantages over the standard oral version, researchers compared them in 11 healthy people. Each subject received three versions of olanzapine 5 mg, about 2 weeks apart: regular olanzapine tablets, olanzapine ODT swallowed, and olanzapine ODT sublingually. For the sublingual form, subjects were encouraged to leave the medicine in their mouth for 15 minutes. The sublingual condition was added to see if pregastric absorption would speed up the effects of ODT.

After taking the dose, 14 samples of blood were drawn over the next 8 hours. Both ODT formulations reached peak concentration a bit earlier than the tablet:

- Tablet: 4.4 hours
- ODT swallowed: 3.5 hours
- ODT sublingual: 3.8 hours

Perhaps more relevant for use in acute agitation, researchers found that at the 10-minute mark, both ODT forms were detectable in subjects' serum, whereas it took 30 minutes for the tablet form to be detectable. There was no statistically significant difference between swallowing the ODT and allowing it to dissolve sublingually (Markowitz JS et al, *J Clin Pharmacol* 2006;46(2):164–171).

The bottom line is that olanzapine ODT is a good choice for rapid control of agitation when patients are willing to take a pill, and it has the advantage of being very difficult to cheek because it dissolves almost instantaneously.

Does Olanzapine ODT Cause Less Weight Gain?

Soon after its release in 2000, the idea began to spread that olanzapine ODT caused less weight gain than the standard tablet. The theory was that the ODT version would have less contact with the appetite-regulating serotonin receptors in the gut. By 2010, there were nine open-label studies and case reports documenting weight loss (half a pound a week, on average) after switching from standard olanzapine to ODT.

However, this is a cautionary tale. Like a lot of ideas in psychiatry, the uncontrolled, open-label studies were positive, but all three randomized, placebo-controlled trials that followed were negative. It's tempting to believe in the open-label studies, since they tell a hopeful story that's easy to understand. The problem is that they don't tell the whole story. Besides the hidden placebo effect, there's a strong publication bias against negative studies. Lots of doctors switched their patients to ODT, but only the handful who saw a drop in weight bothered to publish their observations.

Dissolvable Zolpidem Formulations

Zolpidem (Ambien) comes in three sublingual forms. The standard dose (Edluar) is prescribed as 5 or 10 mg before bed just like zolpidem. The low dose (Intermezzo, 1.75–3.5 mg) is FDA approved for middle-of-the-night awakening when patients have at least 4 hours left to sleep. Then there's Zolpimist, a sprayable liquid that's absorbed under the tongue and through the cheeks and comes in doses equivalent to standard zolpidem. All of these are promoted for their rapid action, but in reality their serum levels take about as long to peak (1 hour Tmax) as regular zolpidem.

Can Patients Have Allergic Reactions to Inactive Ingredients?

The short answer: definitely. A team of researchers at Brigham and Women's Hospital recently published the first comprehensive review of excipients and their potential for adverse reactions. The paper is interesting in a variety of ways. First of all, it's surprising how many inactive ingredients are used in the world of pills. The average pill, they found, is made up of 75% inactive ingredients, with an average of 8.8 excipients present.

How common are allergies to inactive ingredients? 90% of oral medications have at least one excipient that has been reported to cause adverse reactions in sensitive patients. Common culprits found in pills include lactose (present in 45% of oral drugs), peanut oil (often found in valproic acid), gluten (in 18% of drugs), and chemical dyes (Reker D et al, *Sci Transl Med* 2019;11(483):eaau6753).

If you have patients with sensitivities to lactose, peanuts, gluten, or chemical dyes, make sure they know to work with their pharmacist in identifying pills that may contain these products.

The Myth of the "Expired Pill"

If a medication expires in March 2028, that means it will remain stable until at least March 2028, but the medication won't necessarily expire then—it could remain active for many years after that. The reason for this confusion has to do with a loophole in the FDA regulations. Drug manufacturers are required to state how long a drug remained stable in their testing before releasing it to the public, but they aren't required to carry on that testing to the point of expiration. That would be a long time, and pharmaceutical companies are understandably impatient to bring their products to market. That's why the typical expiration date for most medications is 1 year out, but most remain "good" for decades when tested by independent labs. "Good" means that the medication retains 90% of its dosage.

In one study, eight long-expired medications with 15 different active ingredients were discovered in a retail pharmacy in their original, unopened containers. All had "expired" 28 to 40 years prior to analysis. Researchers chemically analyzed the pills and found that 12 of the 14 drug compounds tested (86%) were present in concentrations of at least 90% of the labeled amounts—and two registered at 110% concentration, even higher than the labeled levels (Cantrell L et al, *Arch Intern Med* 2012;172(21):1685–1687).

There are many more formulations of drugs to choose from, but you'll have a better sense of how to use them after we describe how they are absorbed and metabolized in the next two chapters. Then we'll get into the XRs, transdermals, injectables, and other creative formulations that have blossomed in recent years.

CHAPTER 3

GI Absorption, Distribution, and the Blood-Brain Barrier

IN THIS CHAPTER, WE'LL FOCUS on the most common way that our patients take their medications: by mouth, or "PO" (an abbreviation of the Latin "per os," meaning by mouth). When a patient puts a pill or capsule in their mouth, it begins a process through which the molecules get absorbed into the body and transported to the organ of interest—which, for our patients, is the brain.

To start with an overview, the GI tract is essentially a long tube lined with an absorptive mucous membrane. The tube is divided conceptually into different sections, which have different shapes and are specialized to do different things. As drugs get propelled through the tube, the carriers (capsules or tablets) disintegrate, liberating the drug molecules. These molecules are small enough to pass through cell membranes, which they do as they make direct contact with the gut mucosa. Most drugs that we use are lipophilic, meaning that they have no ionic charge. Only lipophilic drugs diffuse easily through cell membranes in the gut. Once through this epithelium, the drug molecules diffuse into the capillaries, which transport them into arteries. From there, they travel to the organs.

The Details of GI Drug Absorption

Pills gradually move through the entire GI system—the mouth, the esophagus, the stomach, the small intestine, the large intestine, and finally the rectum. For most of the drugs we prescribe, no meaningful absorption occurs in the mouth, as the pills spend very little time there. Nor does the stomach do much absorption; instead, it grinds and shoots acid at the pills, helping them disintegrate. Most actual absorption doesn't occur until the drugs reach the small intestine, an organ that is specialized for this task.

The small intestine contains millions of villi and microvilli in its folds, providing an absorptive area about the size of a tennis court. Now that's a lot of absorption.

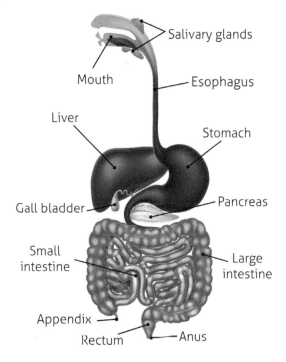

FIGURE 3-1. The GI System

Once drugs are absorbed by the GI tract, they go into the hepatic portal circulation to the liver. This delay before delivery to the target tissues is famously known as the "first-pass effect" because drugs pass first through the liver en route to the heart. Depending on the drug, the liver may metabolize well over 50% of the active ingredients before they arrive at the brain.

There are, however, two regions of the GI tract that drain into vessels that go directly to the heart, bypassing the greedy liver: the sublingual area (under the tongue) and the rectal area. When administered sublingually or rectally, drugs can get to work faster and in higher concentrations. We prescribe drugs this way when rapid onset of action is crucial. Sublingual nitroglycerin, for instance, quickly relieves cardiac anginal pain, hopefully preventing a heart attack. More relevant to psychiatry, sublingual alprazolam quickly relieves the anxiety of panic attacks, and sublingual zolpidem (Edluar and Intermezzo) can be taken in the middle of the night for insomnia. Theoretically, most drugs can be administered sublingually, but some dissolve too slowly or taste too bitter to make this a good option.

Drug Absorption After Bariatric Surgery

There are two main types of bariatric surgery: gastric bypass (Roux-en-Y), in which the stomach is made very small and is attached to the middle part of the small intestine, bypassing the duodenum; and vertical-sleeve gastrectomy, in which much of the stomach is removed, leaving a banana-shaped sleeve that connects directly to the duodenum. While both types of surgery can impair medication absorption, the gastric bypass is the worse actor, since it bypasses part of the intestine where drug absorption occurs.

After bariatric surgery, modified-release (MR) formulations (eg, extended release, controlled release) pose the main challenges because they don't spend enough time in the shortened GI tract to get fully absorbed. These include a few drugs that don't broadcast their MR design: desvenlafaxine (Pristiq), duloxetine (Cymbalta), levomilnacipran (Fetzima), and paliperidone (Invega). Some immediate-release medications can also see a drop in their absorption, like fluoxetine, paroxetine, sertraline, amitriptyline, lamotrigine, olanzapine, and quetiapine. On the other hand, lithium can rise to toxic levels as the patient loses weight after the surgery.

The solution is to switch to immediate-release formulations or, better yet, sublingual, transdermal, or liquid formulations. If the medication is critical to the patient's stability, you may want to check their serum level before and after the bariatric surgery. Serum lab tests are available for most medications and cost $20–$50.

These changes in absorption usually stabilize after 6 months as the GI tract adapts to its new anatomy. At that point, you can slowly revert to the patient's presurgical regimen, checking response and serum levels as you go.

From the GI Tract to the Brain

The remaining active molecules leave the liver through the hepatic vein and then travel through the circulatory system in the following order: the inferior vena cava, the heart's right atrium and ventricle, the pulmonary artery into the lungs, the pulmonary vein to the left atrium and left ventricle. From the left ventricle, blood is pumped into the aorta and onward to systemic circulation.

As our patients' psychotropic-enriched blood is propelled out of the left ventricle and into the ascending aorta, it branches into the left and right common carotids (the right carotid actually branches out of another artery, but close enough). The internal carotid arteries branch off from the common carotids, and these supply blood to the middle and front portions of the brain. The posterior part of the brain is supplied by a more complicated set of arteries, including the vertebral and basilar arteries.

Volume of Distribution

Now is when we have to introduce the somewhat confusing topic of volume of distribution (Vd). It's worth learning, because it has a lot of implications for how we dose medications, especially in patients who are elderly and/or overweight.

The Vd is a measure of how widely a drug is distributed throughout the entire body, as opposed to how much is in the bloodstream alone. It is defined according to the equation:

$$Vd = \frac{\text{Total amount of drug in the body}}{\text{Concentration of drug in the bloodstream}}$$

The concept of Vd has confused medical students through the ages, because a "high volume of distribution" sounds like it should mean that there's a lot of medication around, giving it a strong effect. However, if you take a close look at the equation, you'll see that the opposite is true. A high Vd means that there is relatively little drug in the bloodstream, so less is available to accomplish its therapeutic task. On the other hand, a low Vd means that relatively more medication is available in the blood.

So where does all this drug go if it's not in the bloodstream? Primarily into the adipose tissue. Most drugs dissolve in fatty tissue because they are lipophilic. A typical normal-weight person has a 4:1 ratio of lean to adipose tissue (about 80% lean weight vs 20% fat weight). An obese person (defined as having a body mass index of over 30) has a lean-to-fat ratio closer to 3:2, or 60% lean vs 40% fat (Barras M and Legg A, *Aust Prescr*

2017;40(5):189–193). If there's more fat in the body, lipophilic drugs will be drawn into those fat stores, which means less of the drug is available to have an effect. However, over the ensuing hours or days, the fat stores get saturated and the drug is gradually released back into the bloodstream.

How does knowing this affect your prescribing? In patients with more adipose tissue, the initial doses of a medication may need to be higher to have an effect. This is particularly relevant when treating acute anxiety or agitation. Benzodiazepines and antipsychotics may need to be dosed higher in obese individuals to get around the high volume of distribution. However, over time, with repeated dosing, an equilibrium between fat and bloodstream is reached and you can generally decrease the dose back to normal.

Aside from obese patients, other people with relatively more adipose tissue include the elderly, who lose lean body mass and therefore may have significant fat stores even if they are underweight. We'll talk more about drug metabolism in the elderly in Chapter 18, but the bottom line is the first dose of an antianxiety medication may need to be relatively higher than you'd expect, followed by lower dosing as you continue the medication.

While lipid solubility may lower the initial serum levels of a drug, it has a very different effect at the blood-brain barrier. Here, lipid-soluble medications enter the lipid-rich brain more rapidly, which is why benzodiazepines that are highly lipid soluble have a more rapid onset of action.

The Blood-Brain Barrier

At this point we have our drugs in the brain's neighborhood, but how do they actually make it to the neurons where we want them to be? As in the rest of the body, arteries turn into narrow arterioles and then into capillaries, and medications must squeeze between the endothelial cells lining the capillaries in order to make it into the tissue. But in the brain, this vasculature "switches from delivery route to security system," in the words of *The Scientist.*

This is the blood-brain barrier (BBB), and it prevents over 90% of drugs from entering the brain. There are various mechanisms that accomplish this, such as proteins that cause tight junctions between endothelial cells, and efflux transport cells that oust drugs out of the endothelium and back into the bloodstream, like bouncers keeping the riffraff out of a nightclub.

The BBB is one of the reasons that it is difficult to develop new psychiatric drugs. Generally, the lucky few drugs that can make it into the brain share a couple of qualities: They are pretty small molecules, and they are very lipid soluble. Two of the original drugs that fit these criteria are morphine and heroin, which were often used to treat depression and anxiety before 1950. The antidepressants that replaced them are also small and lipid soluble.

Because neither serotonin nor dopamine can cross the BBB, we cannot use pure neurotransmitters to treat brain illness. In order to affect serotonin levels, we must do so indirectly by creating drugs that are small enough to get inside the brain, where they can increase the supply of serotonin by interfering with reuptake.

This is also why we can't treat Parkinson's disease (caused by a dopamine deficiency) by giving pure dopamine, which doesn't cross the BBB. Instead, we give dopamine's precursor, levodopa, which can enter the brain and then be metabolized to dopamine. Sinemet, a common Parkinson's treatment, is actually a combination of levodopa and carbidopa; carbidopa is added to prevent the levodopa from being degraded too much before it enters the brain, which minimizes peripheral side effects.

That's how the journey looks, but to troubleshoot your patient's meds and dose them correctly, you'll need to know how the journey is measured. In the next chapter, we'll look at how fast medications get in and out of the system and how high their levels go.

CHAPTER 4

Basic Pharmacokinetics: Onset, Duration, and Half-Life

PHARMACOKINETICS REFERS TO HOW DRUGS move through the body and what makes their serum levels go high or low. Pharmacodynamics, on the other hand, refers to a drug's therapeutic and adverse effects. The two are sometimes distinguished in the following way: Pharmacokinetics is what the body does to the drug, whereas pharmacodynamics is what the drug does to the body. In this chapter, we'll review the need-to-know material on pharmacokinetics that will guide your medication decisions.

Tmax, Cmax, and Onset of Action

After a patient swallows a pill, the drug is absorbed and rises fairly quickly to a peak concentration, termed "Cmax." The time required for a particular drug to reach Cmax is called its "Tmax." Note that Tmax is not the same thing as onset of action. For example, sildenafil (Viagra) takes about an hour to reach Cmax, but its onset of action is 20–30 minutes. This is because most drugs start to affect the body at concentrations lower than their maximum eventual concentrations. For sildenafil, the effective concentration is attained well before Cmax (this is true for benzodiazepines as well).

After reaching Cmax, the concentration gradually falls, eventually reaching a "Cmin," or trough concentration, just before the next dose is taken. Graphically, the best way to comprehend these concepts is to look at a concentration-time curve, which is printed in the *Physician's Desk Reference (PDR)* for most drugs. It shows how the amount of a single dose of a drug in the blood varies over time:

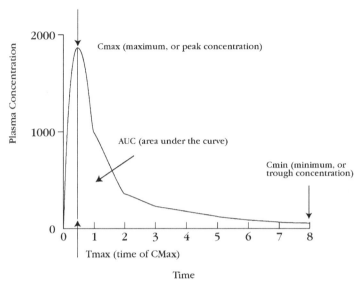

FIGURE 4-1. Concentration-Time Curve

The area under the curve (AUC) is a measure of the total amount of drug absorbed by the body over time, and it's often used by drug reps to promote modified-release (MR) formulations of drugs. They may show you such curves to prove that a once-a-day MR formulation leads to an AUC comparable to BID or TID dosing of the instant-release formulation. We'll scrutinize the value of MR compounds more closely in Chapter 5.

Half-Life

The half-life is the time required for half of a drug to leave your patient's body. Five is the magic number: It takes 5 half-lives for a drug to be completely cleared from the patient's system. Conversely, it takes 5 half-lives after a patient starts taking a drug for it to reach a steady state, at which point a blood level is reliable.

Dosing by Half-Life

When a manufacturer releases a new medication, it usually bases the dosing schedule on the half-life. A medication with a 24-hour half-life is dosed once a day (QD); one with a 12-hour half-life is dosed twice a day (BID); and a drug with an 8-hour half-life is dosed three times a day (TID). Over time, clinicians often simplify these schedules to once a day. That makes it easier for patients to follow, but does it compromise the drugs' efficacy?

A few studies have tested this out, comparing daily to twice-daily dosing for antipsychotics and antidepressants with short half-lives. In all cases that we're aware of, the two dosing strategies had the same outcomes. The most likely explanation is that the involved drugs' therapeutic benefits depend on downstream effects like neurotropic factors and receptor adaptation, and the brain doesn't require constant steady-state exposure to the drug to achieve those effects (Yýldýz A and Sachs GS, *J Affect Disord* 2001;66(2–3):199–206).

Once-a-day dosing is more likely to alter a drug's side effects than its therapeutic effects. Sedation improves with evening dosing, a strategy that has been successfully employed with antidepressant doses of trazodone, which can be given entirely at night. Other side effects improve with divided dosing, particularly the ones that worsen as the level peaks: nausea, dizziness, fatigue, orthostasis, and QTc prolongation.

VERDICT

Psychiatric medications with delayed benefits can usually be given once a day without loss of efficacy. This strategy improves some side effects like sedation, but other side effects benefit from spreading out the dose and lowering the drug's peak levels.

The Half-Lives of Stimulants and Sedatives

Stimulants and sedatives are among the few psychiatric medications with immediate effects, so these drugs are usually given in divided doses that follow their half-lives. For example, alprazolam has a half-life of 6–12 hours and is dosed every 6–12 hours. Why the range? Half-lives are not fixed in stone but vary by patient. Ask your patient when they feel the medication start to wear off, and use that to personalize the dosing schedule.

Anything that speeds up drug metabolism will shorten the half-life, necessitating more frequent dosing. Metabolism is speeded up by drug interactions with potent inducers, genetic variations of the "rapid metabolizer" type, and youth. The opposite factors slow down drug metabolism and lengthen the half-life: drug interactions with potent inhibitors, genetic variations of the "poor metabolizer" type, and old age. For example, lamotrigine's half-life is 24 hours, but that stretches to 48 hours with a potent inhibitor like valproate and shrinks to 12 hours with a potent inducer like carbamazepine.

We've listed the half-lives of stimulants and sedatives in the following tables, from the prescribed to the unprescribed (but often taken, like caffeine). Here are a few trends to pay attention to. When selecting a sleep medication, a short half-life option like zaleplon (Sonata) is less likely to cause problems with memory or coordination the next morning. Zaleplon's half-life is 1 hour, which is why the FDA allows it to be taken a little later than other hypnotics (specifically, after the patient has gone to bed and has experienced difficulty falling asleep instead of restricting the dose to before bed).

You'll notice that benzodiazepines are often dosed more frequently than their half-lives would suggest. This is because their duration of action

TABLE 4-1. Stimulant Half-Lives

Stimulant	Half-Life	Dosing Schedule
Caffeine	3–4 hr	Varies
Methylphenidate and dexmethylphenidate	3 hr	TID
Amphetamine salts and dextroamphetamine	10–14 hr	BID
Modafinil and armodafinil	15 hr	QAM

TABLE 4-2. Benzodiazepine Half-Lives

Benzo	Half-Life	Half-Life of Active Metabolites	Dosing Schedule	Dose Equivalent to Clonazepam 1 mg
Triazolam	2–6 hr	None	QHS	0.5–1 mg
Oxazepam	4–15 hr	None	TID–QID	60 mg
Temazepam	8–22 hr	None	QHS	30–60 mg
Alprazolam	6–12 hr	None	BID–TID	1–2 mg
Lorazepam	10–20 hr	None	BID–TID	2–4 mg
Estazolam	10–24 hr	None	QHS	2–4 mg
Clonazepam	1–2 days	None	BID	1 mg
Quazepam	2–3 days	1–6 days	QHS	30–40 mg
Diazepam	1–4 days	1–8 days	BID–TID	20 mg
Clorazepate	< 30 min	2–8 days	BID–QID	30 mg
Chlordiazepoxide	0.5–2 days	2–8 days	BID–QID	50 mg
Flurazepam	2–3 hr	2–10 days	QHS	30–60 mg

TABLE 4-3. Sedative-Hypnotic Half-Lives

Sedative	Half-Life	Tmax
Melatonin	40–60 min	15–30 min
Ramelteon (Rozerem)	1–2 hr	45 min
Zaleplon (Sonata)	1.5 hr	1 hr
Zolpidem (Ambien)	2.5 hr	1.6 hr
Prazosin	2.5 hr	1 hr
Diphenhydramine (Benadryl)	2–4 hr	2 hr
Eszopiclone (Lunesta)	6 hr	1 hr
Chloral hydrate	8–10 hr	30 min
Doxylamine (Unisom)	10 hr	1.5–2.5 hr
Trazodone	5–9 hr	1–2 hr
Suvorexant (Belsomra)	15 hr	2 hr
Lemborexant (Dayvigo)	18 hr	1–3 hr
Hydroxyzine	20 hr	2 hr
Doxepin (Silenor)	15–30 hr	3.5 hr

depends on their levels in the CNS, not in the bloodstream. Some benzodiazepines (the more lipophilic or "fat-loving" ones) get into the CNS faster, like diazepam and the ones that are approved for sleep (estazolam, flurazepam, quazepam, temazepam, and triazolam). That means they work faster, but this rapid onset of action also makes them more likely to cause amnesia and addiction. If you have to use a benzo in a patient with a history of addiction, consider one with a slower onset like lorazepam or—the slowest of all—oxazepam.

Several benzodiazepines have "effective half-lives" that are longer than their actual half-life. This is because they are converted into other active benzos through hepatic enzymes, and these active metabolites extend the original medications' effective half-lives by several days. Chlordiazepoxide and diazepam are metabolized into oxazepam and nordiazepam, and diazepam is further dismantled into temazepam. This kind of metabolic buildup can be dangerous in the elderly, who have trouble clearing out all these metabolites. On the other hand, having active metabolites can be beneficial in situations like alcohol detox treatment, because those metabolites prevent breakthrough withdrawal symptoms between doses.

Dosing schedules are more critical with fast-acting medications, but half-life is only a rough guide to dosing frequency. Some drugs need more frequent administration than their half-life suggests because they don't spend as much time in the CNS as they do in the bloodstream.

Short Half-Lives and Drug Discontinuation

One risk with short half-life drugs is that they cause withdrawal symptoms as they quickly exit the body. This is a particular problem with benzodiazepines and serotonergic antidepressants like SSRIs and SNRIs. The syndromes themselves are quite awful, and raise fears of addiction that cause some patients to avoid psychiatric medications altogether.

About half of patients experience withdrawal problems from SSRIs and SNRIs, including dizziness, electric shock sensations, ear ringing, headache, and fatigue, as well as mood and anxiety symptoms that can make it look like they are relapsing back into depression.

The severity of serotonin withdrawal generally falls right in line with the half-life, with one exception: paroxetine (Paxil). This SSRI ranks right beside venlafaxine as having the most notorious withdrawal problems, but its 20-hour half-life is 3–4 times longer than venlafaxine's brief 5 hours. The reason is that paroxetine slows down its own metabolism by inhibiting the enzyme that metabolizes it (CYP2D6). When your patient stops paroxetine, this enzyme revs back up, effectively shortening the half-life and hastening the withdrawal (Fava GA and Grandi S, *J Clin Psychopharmacol* 1995;15(5):374–375).

There are two ways to manage withdrawal syndromes. You can either taper the original drug slowly (eg, over several months), or switch to a long half-life drug, such as fluoxetine for serotonin withdrawal syndrome or diazepam for the benzodiazepines. You may still need to taper off the old drug as you add in the long half-life version because the new medication won't bind to the receptor in exactly the same way.

What about changing to a modified-release (MR) version to prevent withdrawal? This might sound like a good idea, but it will only change the rate of absorption, not of excretion, so MRs don't actually lengthen the half-life. However, if you factor in the delay between swallowing the pill and excreting it, they do effectively slow down the final clearance of the drug (ie, the effective half-life), but the difference is usually not enough to ease a withdrawal syndrome.

The Pros and Cons of a Long Half-Life

Long half-life drugs stay a while, which is a plus for patients who miss occasional doses (ie, most patients). On the other hand, these extended stays are a liability when drug interactions are involved, as when you have to wait for 5 half-lives to pass to avoid drug interactions before starting an MAOI. For fluoxetine, the wait is 6 weeks, vortioxetine is 2 weeks, and for most other antidepressants it is 3–5 days.

Fluoxetine's lingering half-life can also cause a problem when it's used in bipolar disorder in the form of olanzapine/fluoxetine combination (OFC or Symbyax). In bipolar depression, fluoxetine is supposed to be taken along with olanzapine to counteract the SSRI's pro-manic effects. When

Half-Lives in Action: Modafinil vs Armodafinil

Modafinil (Provigil) and armodafinil (Nuvigil) are wakefulness-promoting medications that are used off label in psychiatry for depression, fatigue, and ADHD. Like many medications, modafinil is actually two chemicals that are mirror images of each other, called enantiomers. They are armodafinil and S-modafinil, and Nuvigil is pure armodafinil. These two enantiomers have similar potencies but different half-lives, which is why there is no simple way to convert from modafinil to armodafinil. Armodafinil's half-life is 15 hours, while S-modafinil's is 4–5 hours. This means that when your patient takes modafinil (a 50/50 mix of the two enantiomers), they will get a bigger effect in the first half of the day, but that will wear off as the short-acting S-modafinil quickly tapers out. In contrast, armodafinil (Nuvigil) delivers steadier levels throughout the day.

VERDICT

Most patients prefer the smoother, longer-lasting armodafinil (Nuvigil), but those who need more help in the morning or have insomnia on the drug should try modafinil (Provigil).

TABLE 4-4. Short Half-Life Drugs

Class	Half-Life (hours)	Relevance
SSRIs	Fluvoxamine (15), paroxetine (15–21)	Higher risk of withdrawal syndrome
SNRIs	Venlafaxine (5), milnacipran (Savella) (8), desvenlafaxine* (Pristiq) (11), duloxetine* (12), levomilnacipran* (Fetzima) (12)	Higher risk of withdrawal syndrome
Other antidepressants	Nefazodone (2–4), amoxapine (8), bupropion (14)	Bupropion IR should be divided TID to avoid seizures; nefazodone and amoxapine can be given BID or QHS; amoxapine is the only tricyclic with a short half-life
MAOIs	Tranylcypromine (2), isocarboxazid (2–4), phenelzine (12), selegiline patch (EMSAM) (22), selegiline oral (2–10)	Most MAOIs are dosed BID, and selegiline patch is dosed QD
Buspirone	2–3	Can be dosed BID or TID
Anticonvulsants	Gabapentin (6), pregabalin (6), tiagabine (8), oxcarbazepine (7–20), carbamazepine (12–17), valproate (9–16)	Carbamazepine and valproate should be dosed BID; oxcarbazepine's half-life is prolonged from 1–5 to 7–20 hr by its active metabolite, MHD
Antipsychotics	Loxapine (3), quetiapine (7), ziprasidone (7), thioridazine (8), perphenazine (10), clozapine (12), fluphenazine (15)	Short half-life antipsychotics can be dosed once a day to improve adherence
Tardive dyskinesia	Deutetrabenazine (Austedo) (9)	Deutetrabenazine needs to be dosed BID to reduce the risk of QTc prolongation; valbenazine has a longer half-life and is dosed QHS, unless drug interactions or genetic factors cause its half-life to shorten (see Chapter 20)
Sexual	Bremelanotide (Vyleesi) (3), flibanserin (Addyi) (6), sildenafil (Viagra) (4), vardenafil (Levitra) (5)	The 18-hour half-life of tadalafil (Cialis) is longer than the others, allowing a needed window of spontaneity

*These antidepressants can be dosed QD because they were originally released, and are only available, as XR formulations

TABLE 4-5. Long Half-Life Drugs

Class	Half-Life	Relevance
Antidepressants	Vortioxetine (3 days), protriptyline (2–8 days), fluoxetine (1–4 days; active metabolite 7–10 days)	Fluoxetine is the SSRI with the lowest withdrawal risk; protriptyline is the only tricyclic with a long half-life
Antipsychotics	Cariprazine (2–4 days; active metabolites up to 3 weeks), aripiprazole (3 days), brexpiprazole (4 days), pimozide (4–5 days), pimavanserin (2 days; active metabolite 8 days)	These antipsychotics are good choices for patients who miss doses
Other	Disulfiram (2–3 days), memantine (2–3 days), donepezil (3 days), levothyroxine (6–7 days)	Disulfiram's alcohol interactions persist for up to 2 weeks after it is stopped

OFC is stopped, the olanzapine leaves quickly over 5 days, but fluoxetine lingers for over a month. A safer approach is to stop fluoxetine first and then taper off the olanzapine.

Most psychotropics have half-lives in the medium range, around 24 hours. It's the ones with short and long half-lives that you need to know, and we've listed them in tables 4-4 and 4-5 with practical tips on how their half-lives inform their use.

How Lithium Reaches Steady State in 5 Half-Lives

Have you ever wondered what "steady state" actually means, why it takes 5 half-lives to achieve it, and what makes it the right time to get an accurate blood level? The answer is not as simple as you might think. A common misconception about steady state is that it means the serum drug levels are the same throughout the day. Not true. Steady state means your body is eliminating the drug at the same overall rate as you are ingesting it.

To understand how this works, let's look at the example of starting a patient on lithium, a drug that requires periodic monitoring to ensure an adequate dose and prevent toxicity. The half-life of lithium is about 24 hours. Let's assume we start our patient on 600 mg QD on day 1 (see "Day 1 Max" in the chart below). 24 hours later, just before his second dose on day 2, the amount left in his body is 300 mg ("Day 2 Min"), because 24 hours (one half-life) have passed; therefore, the patient has excreted half of the initial amount. He then swallows another 600 mg for his day 2 dose, resulting in a day 2 max of 300 mg + 600 mg = 900 mg. On day 3, he starts the day with half of 900 mg, or 450 mg, and after his 600 mg dose he has 1050 mg. And so on. As you can see, with each passing day, the blood levels—both peak and trough—become more and more predictable. They still fluctuate by 600 mg a day, but the peak and trough are relatively stable.

And this explains why we wait 5 half-lives before drawing a blood level. At day 2, the trough blood level would be 300, and at day 3, it would be 450. There's a big difference between 300 mg and 450 mg, which shows why drawing blood levels too early yields unreliable results. However, a blood level draw at day 5 (562) is not much different from day 7 (590), which in turn will not be much different from the result on day 300, as long as the dose stays at 600 mg. Eventually, a limit is reached, with the peak hovering around 1200 and the trough around 600.

Body Content of Lithium in Milligrams	Day 1	Day 2		Day 3		Day 4	
	Max	Min	Max	Min	Max	Min	Max
	600	300	900	450	1050	525	1125
	Day 5		Day 6		Day 7		
	Min	Max	Min	Max	Min	Max	
	562	1162	581	1181	590	1190	

FIGURE 4-2. How Lithium Rises When Dosed 600 mg QHS

VERDICT

It takes 5 half-lives to achieve steady state, and that's how long you need to wait before checking a serum level on drugs like lithium, valproate, or carbamazepine. If you check any earlier, your trough level will underestimate the actual level that the patient will achieve after steady state.

Do Drugs With Long Half-Lives Take Longer to Work?

There's a strange myth floating around that drugs with long half-lives take longer to work than drugs with short half-lives. Apparently, this comes from misinterpreting the meaning of steady state. It's true that long half-life meds take longer to get to steady state. For example, fluoxetine, in concert with its norfluoxetine metabolite, has a half-life of about 2 weeks and takes 2 ½ months to reach steady state. Nonetheless, fluoxetine works just as quickly as short half-life antidepressants (Gelenberg AJ and Chesen CL, *J Clin Psychiatry* 2000;61(10):712–721). Evidently, serotonin receptors aren't waiting around for fluoxetine to reach steady state. Still, it can take time for the rising level to reach an effective dosage (eg, OCD often requires higher doses of SSRIs). While the slow rise in serum levels doesn't lower the efficacy, it may cause some side effects to build up as the levels rise over weeks or months, sometimes requiring a dose adjustment to improve tolerability.

Linear vs Nonlinear Pharmacokinetics

Drugs with linear pharmacokinetics rise predictably along a straight line (this is sometimes called "first-order pharmacokinetics"). When you double the dose, the serum level doubles. Most psychiatric medications operate this way, but there are a few that follow the unwieldy rules of nonlinear pharmacokinetics, rising faster or slower than expected.

Three SSRIs rise faster than expected: fluoxetine, fluvoxamine, and paroxetine. These three inhibit their own metabolism after a few days, effectively slowing their excretion and stretching their half-lives. The other three nonlinear meds rise slower than expected, and they are all anticonvulsants: carbamazepine, valproate, and gabapentin.

Each of these anticonvulsants has a different reason for its slow rise. Carbamazepine induces its own metabolism, hastening its excretion and shortening its half-life. This effect revs up gradually over 2–4 weeks, which is why carbamazepine levels need to be rechecked 1–2 months after starting it. Valproate has trouble getting into the serum because it binds to proteins that render it therapeutically inactive. This is particularly true at the lower levels (eg, < 50 mcg/mL), so you can expect dose changes to make a more dramatic difference when the patient's valproate level is in the higher range. Gabapentin's pattern is the opposite. It rises quickly at first and then slows down. Gabapentin saturates the transporters that absorb it in the small intestine, causing its levels to rise at a snail's pace when the dose goes above the saturation point (around 900 mg/day). From there, its absorption trickles down. At 900 mg/day, 60% is absorbed; at 1200 mg/day, it drops to 50%; and at 3000 mg/day, only 30% of the gabapentin you've prescribed is actually getting into the patient's system.

VERDICT

Carbamazepine's levels will drop after 1–2 months. For valproate, small dose changes can have big effects once the level is beyond 50 mcg/mL. High doses of gabapentin are not as big as they seem once you get beyond 900 mg/day.

Potency vs Effectiveness

The term "potency" often confuses patients, and occasionally clinicians as well. In general, potency refers to a drug's power per unit, or the amount of pharmacological activity per milligram. This issue sometimes comes up when we switch from one medication to another. For example, switching from 20 mg of fluoxetine to 150 mg of venlafaxine XR sometimes causes patients to wonder if we are trying to overdose them. Conversely (and probably more relevant to patient safety), when we switch from, say, 100 mg of sertraline to 20 mg of citalopram, some patients may think that they are being underdosed and may then increase their doses between visits if they do not see a rapid improvement.

VERDICT

Clarify the difference between potency and dose for patients before switching medications. For benzodiazepines, the relative potencies are listed in Table 4-2 on page 24 and can be used to guide the transition from one benzo to another.

Now that you understand how to shift the manual gears of pharmacokinetics, we'll look at something closer to an automatic transmission: the modified release.

CHAPTER 5

Modified-Release Medications: XR, CR, ER, and Beyond

ONCE-A-DAY DOSING IS HARD ENOUGH, and twice a day is a little worse, but adherence takes a sharp decline when the dosing schedule jumps to three or four times a day. Modified-release formulations were developed in the 1960s to solve this problem, and they've become increasingly sophisticated in the decades since.

Modified-release medications go by many names—controlled, extended, prolonged, delayed, slow, and sustained—but there are really only two categories: sustained release and delayed release. As their names imply, sustained-release pills smooth out the serum levels by releasing the medication at a steady rate. Delayed-release pills don't get absorbed until they've traveled to a specific site in the gut, hence "delaying" their release. To avoid confusion, we'll use the term modified release (MR) throughout this book to refer to all these formulations and distinguish them from their immediate-release (IR) forbearers.

IR medications dissolve rapidly in the GI tract and are absorbed within an hour or two. Their serum concentrations spike quickly and then fall back down, leading to low trough levels before the next dose. Those ups and downs in serum levels can cause side effects or efficacy problems. For example, bupropion can increase the risk of seizures if the serum level peaks too high, IR stimulants can lose efficacy in the afternoon, and the rise and fall of haloperidol levels increases the likelihood of dystonic reactions.

How MR Medications Work

Modified-release mechanisms come in many variations, and these mechanisms have gotten more complex and sophisticated since the first one—Dexedrine Spansules—was released in 1952. We don't need to know the gory details of their underlying physics, but it's useful to at least get an overview and learn a few common examples in depth.

There are generally three release mechanisms. In *dissolution control,* the medication is released as the outer coating dissolves (Dexedrine Spansules, Seroquel XR, Mydayis, and Adhansia). In *diffusion control,* the medicine slowly diffuses out of a semipermeable membrane (Effexor XR capsules, Wellbutrin XL, and Focalin XR). And in *osmotic-release* pills, the medicine is pushed out by a tiny pump that's powered by the osmotic flow of water across a semipermeable membrane (Concerta, Invega, and Effexor XR tablets). Often, a formulation will combine several of these technologies.

Pros and Cons of Modified-Release Medications

With their convenient dosing and lower rates of side effects, the pros usually outweigh the cons for MRs. But there are situations where the instant release is preferred, such as in the first 6 months after bariatric surgery when the truncated GI tract is unable to fully absorb an MR medication.

TABLE 5-1. Modified-Release Medications: Pros and Cons

Pros	Cons
Less frequent dosing	Less flexible dosing
Smoother plasma levels	Inconsistent absorption, particularly after bariatric surgery
Fewer adverse effects	Prolongation of adverse effects
Lower abuse potential	Higher risk of accidental overdose with MR opioids and benzos
Some are available as easy-to-swallow liquids or chews (Quillivant XR liquid and QuilliChew ER) or capsules that can be opened and sprinkled	Most come as large pills that are difficult to swallow
	Higher cost

Dosing Convenience

MR mechanisms offer convenient dosing, but some patients prefer the flexibility of immediate release. That's particularly true with stimulants and benzos. Most of us have patients with ADHD who, for example, prefer methylphenidate IR over MR versions such as Concerta. The IR stimulant allows them to take more or fewer pills depending on the concentration demands of the day.

Splitting and Crushing

Most MR medications can't be split or crushed without disrupting the integrity of the time-release mechanism. This makes it more difficult to titrate or taper doses of these drugs in small increments. However, a few MR medications come as capsules that can be opened and partially sprinkled out because each bead inside the capsule has its own time-release mechanism. Some medications are on both lists because you can sprinkle them but you can't crush them.

TABLE 5-2. MR Medications That Can Be Opened or Sprinkled

Adderall XR, Mydayis, Dexedrine Spansules
Carbamazepine XR (Equetro, Carbatrol, Tegretol XR)
Depakote sprinkles
Dexmethylphenidate XR (Focalin XR)
Duloxetine sprinkles
Namenda XR, Namzaric
Ritalin LA, Aptensio XR, Jornay PM, Metadate CD, Adhansia XR
Topiramate (all forms including IR)
Venlafaxine XR
Viloxazine ER (Qelbree)
Vyvanse

TABLE 5-3. The Do Not Crush List

Abilify MyCite kit
Adderall XR, Adzenys XR-ODT, Mydayis
Alprazolam XR
Ambien CR, Edluar
Amphetamine ODT (Evekeo ODT)
Bupropion (all forms: IR, XL, SR, Aplenzin, Zyban)
Carbamazepine XR (Equetro, Carbatrol, Tegretol XR)
Clonidine ER (Kapvay)
Concerta, Cotempla XR-ODT, Adhansia XR, Aptensio XR, Jornay PM, Metadate CD, Metadate ER, Methylin ER, Ritalin LA

(table continues)

TABLE 5-3. The Do Not Crush List *(continued)*

Depakene, Depakote, Depakote ER
Desvenlafaxine (Pristiq, Khedezla)
Deutetrabenazine (Austedo)
Dexmethylphenidate XR (Focalin XR)
Donepezil (Aricept) 23 mg
Duloxetine
Fluoxetine weekly (Prozac Weekly)
Fluvoxamine ER
Gabapentin (Neurontin, Gralise, Horizant)
Galantamine ER (Razadyne ER)
Guanfacine ER (Intuniv)
Lamotrigine XR
Lithium ER (Lithobid) and CR (Eskalith)
Memantine XR (Namenda XR), memantine/donepezil combo (Namzaric)
Metformin XR (Glucophage XR)
Oxcarbazepine XR (Oxtellar XR)
Paliperidone (Invega)
Paroxetine IR, CR, and mesylate forms (Paxil, Pexeva)
Pregabalin CR (Lyrica CR)
Quetiapine XR
Strattera (contents can irritate the eyes)
Topiramate (bad taste if crushed)
Venlafaxine XR
Viloxazine ER (Qelbree)

MR Medications and Side Effects

Some side effects improve with MR mechanisms, particularly those that result from high serum levels (fatigue, dry mouth, and dizziness) or direct irritation of the GI tract (nausea). On the other hand, MRs can cause side effects to last too long. Insomnia on stimulants and morning-after effects with MR hypnotics are two examples. This is why the FDA has a stronger warning about driving in the morning after taking zolpidem CR than they do for zolpidem IR.

MR Medications and Substance Use Disorders

Modified-release mechanisms might reduce the abuse potential of controlled substances because they dampen the reinforcing peaks in the serum level (known as the Cmax). This is true in theory and is supported by a study where subjects with a history of sedative abuse were given blinded samples of alprazolam XR, alprazolam IR, and placebo. When asked if they would be willing to pay cash to have another dose, they answered "yes" for the IR but "no" for the XR and placebo (Mumford GK et al, *Clin Pharmacol Ther* 1995;57(3):356–365).

Patients who are committed to getting high can still overcome the MR obstacle by crushing the pill and snorting or injecting the contents. A possible exception is Vyvanse, which does not become pharmacologically active until it is cleaved in the bloodstream.

On the other hand, MR formulations increase the risk of an accidental overdose by prolonging the effects of the drug. This is well documented with opioids, where MR formulations double the risk of accidental overdose (Chua KP et al, *JAMA Pediatr* 2020;174(2):141–148).

Ghost Pills

The sight of an undigested capsule in their stool is an unpleasant surprise for many patients. However, this "ghost pill" is normal and expected with modified-release capsules that use an osmotic delivery system. The medication is absorbed, but the capsule is excreted intact. A little advance warning helps, so consider informing your patients about the possibility of ghost pills from the following medications: Concerta, carbamazepine XR (Tegretol XR), paliperidone (Invega), and venlafaxine XR tablets (Effexor).

A less alarming phenomenon occurs with diffusion-controlled release mechanisms. Here, parts of the pill may pass into the stool. This can occur with bupropion XL (Wellbutrin XL or Aplenzin), desvenlafaxine tablets (Pristiq), Focalin XR capsules, Ritalin SR tablets, and venlafaxine XR capsules (Effexor).

Specific Modified-Release Medications

Antidepressants

Patients with depression have a hard enough time getting out of bed and brushing their teeth. Expecting them to take a medication multiple times a day is not a recipe for success. MR formulations are helpful here, particularly with the otherwise thrice-daily bupropion and venlafaxine. Three other antidepressants are only available as MRs: desvenlafaxine (Pristiq), duloxetine (Cymbalta), and levomilnacipran (Fetzima). With their 12-hour half-lives, these three would normally be dosed twice a day, but their manufacturers spared our patients that tedium by releasing them exclusively in MR forms.

Bupropion

There are four formulations of bupropion on the market (Table 5-4). All four versions contain the same molecule, of course (bupropion), and there is no difference in antidepressant efficacy among them. As you might expect, the IR version releases all of its medication quickly (its Tmax is quite short at 1.5 hours) followed by progressively more delayed release in the SR and XR. Figure 5-1 on page 40 compares the concentration-time curves of three of the versions (IR, SR, and XL). Wellbutrin IR has a sawtooth pattern, with three Grand Teton–type peaks corresponding to TID dosing; SR has two gentler peaks; and XL has only one broad Appalachian-appearing peak.

Bupropion and Seizure Risk

Do any of the modified-release formulations decrease seizure risk? Possibly, since seizure risk is related to the peak level, and these formulations smooth over those peaks and reduce the risk that patients will take their doses too close together. But the greater player in the seizure risk is the total daily dose.

When bupropion was first released in 1985, it was available in the IR versions only, and the suggested daily maximum dose was 600 mg. The rate of seizures with those liberal dosing limits was an alarming 3%, and the drug was withdrawn from the market in 1986. It returned in 1989 with a more cautious maximum dose of 450 mg. Bupropion's seizure risk fell to 0.4% at 450 mg/day and 0.1% at 300 mg/day—and now it's actually one of the antidepressants least likely to cause seizures. In fact, a 2018 meta-analysis ranked it near the bottom for its epileptogenic effects. In that analysis, clomipramine had the highest risk, followed by amitriptyline, venlafaxine, citalopram, sertraline, trazodone, mirtazapine, paroxetine, bupropion, escitalopram, fluoxetine, and duloxetine (Steinert T and Fröscher W, *Pharmacopsychiatry* 2018;51(4):121–135).

TABLE 5-4. Bupropion Formulations

	Dosages Available (mg)	Max Allowed in a Single Dose	How to Dose 300 mg Daily	Tmax at 300 mg Daily
Bupropion IR	75, 100	150 mg	100 mg TID	1.5 hours
Bupropion SR	100, 150, 200	200 mg	150 mg BID	2.5 hours
Bupropion ER/XL (eg, Forfivo)	150, 300, 450	450 mg	300 mg QAM	5 hours
Bupropion hydrobromide ER (Aplenzin)	174, 348, 522	522 mg	348 mg QAM	5 hours

Let's go through each of the formulations of bupropion and discuss the pros and cons of choosing it for a particular patient:

Bupropion IR: The rationale for starting patients on IR is that you want to see whether they will have any side effects at the lowest exposure possible. Then, when it's clear they tolerate it, you will switch to one of the time-release formulations. We often use this strategy when patients are at risk for significant side effects on bupropion, particularly anxiety, insomnia, and mania. A common sequence would be to start with 75 mg QAM for a few days, then increase to 75 or 100 mg BID, and if they tolerate this you might switch to an MR form, such as SR or XL. Another advantage of the IR medication is that you can cut it in half without disturbing its formulation—good for those patients who are ultra-sensitive to side effects.

Bupropion hydrochloride SR (Wellbutrin SR, Zyban): This early MR formulation reduced bupropion's dosing from TID to BID, but it has largely been supplanted by the once-a-day XL. However, there are a couple reasons to consider the SR. First, the SR is the only version with official FDA approval for smoking cessation, in the form of Zyban, which is identical to generic bupropion SR (target dose 150 mg SR BID). However, bupropion XL also has empirical support for smoking cessation even if it lacks FDA approval (Gray KM et al, *Nicotine Tob Res* 2012;14(2):234–239).

Bupropion IR (100 mg tid)

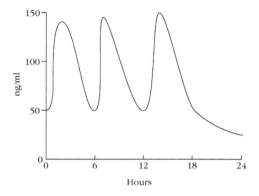

Bupropion SR (150 mg bid)

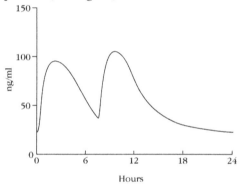

Bupropion XL (300 mg qd)

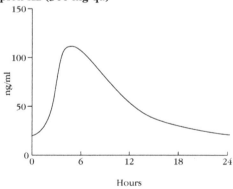

Source: Data from GlaxoSmithKline, Research Triangle Park, NC
Abbreviations: IR = immediate-release, SR = sustained-release, XL = extended-release

FIGURE 5-1. Steady-State Plasma Level Concentrations for Wellbutrin 300 mg/day for IR, SR, and XL Formulations

The other use for the SR is when you are treating depression and you want some sustained blood levels, but you're concerned about insomnia so you don't want to use the XL. In this case you might just prescribe 150–200 mg of the SR in the morning and leave it at that. If you need a higher dose, you can give 150 mg BID with instructions to not take the second dose too late in the day.

Bupropion hydrochloride XL (Wellbutrin XL, Forfivo): Bupropion XL is the favorite of many psychiatrists and their patients because you can safely give the entire effective dose once a day in the morning. Yes, you can go all the way up to 450 mg in a single dose, and the cleverly named Forfivo brand allows you to give 450 mg in a single pill (get it? 4-5-O).

Bupropion hydrobromide XL (Aplenzin): This formulation has similar pharmacokinetics to the previous XL and the same once-a-day dosing, but a different binding agent: hydrobromide instead of hydrochloride. The hydrobromide reduces bupropion's absorption, which is why Aplenzin is packaged in higher doses, each of which is equivalent to small, medium, and large bupropion (174 mg Aplenzin = 150 mg bupropion, 348 mg = 300 mg, and 522 mg = 450 mg). There is no advantage to prescribing Aplenzin, and in fact there is a debatable disadvantage because the bromide that it is packaged with has been linked to various side effects, such as sexual dysfunction and thyroid disorders (Shader RI, *J Clin Psychopharmacol* 2009;29(4):317–318).

VERDICT

Bupropion is probably safer and better tolerated in its modified-release forms. The immediate release comes in a lower dose (75 mg) that's useful for slow titrations in sensitive patients, such as those with anxiety or bipolar disorder, or the very young or very old. Most of the time, bupropion hydrochloride XL is the preferred form.

Venlafaxine XR

Venlafaxine was one of the first MR drugs to capture the imagination of psychiatrists and represents a good success story for MR versions of drugs. Some of you may recall that when Effexor was first introduced in 1995, it was nicknamed "side effexor" because of a harsh combination of nausea, daytime sedation, and nighttime insomnia. In 1997, Effexor XR was introduced, and it was tolerated so much better that it became one of the most widely prescribed antidepressants (Entsuah R and Chitra R,

Psychopharmacol Bull 1997;33(4):671–676). The XR version also simplified the regimen from TID to QD.

The XR capsule is packed with coated spheroids that slowly release their contents as they diffuse through the membrane. A second MR—venlafaxine ER—was released in 2008 with a different mechanism, delivering the drug through an osmotic tablet. The XR and ER formulations have similar pharmacokinetics, but the ER tablets are more expensive.

VERDICT

Venlafaxine XR is a significant improvement over the IR form and less expensive than venlafaxine ER.

Paroxetine

Paroxetine CR has a geomatrix coating that allows the tablet to pass through the stomach unaltered. This means that most of it is absorbed in the small intestine where there are fewer serotonin 5HT-3 receptors, theoretically causing less serotonergic nausea. The early clinical trials comparing paroxetine IR with CR found that fewer patients reported nausea during the first week on CR (14%) than IR (23%). However, by week 2, there were no significant differences in nausea rates between the formulations (Golden RN et al, *J Clin Psychiatry* 2002;63(7):577–584).

VERDICT

Paroxetine CR has only mild advantages over the IR form.

Fluoxetine Weekly

Fluoxetine weekly is a delayed-release version of the antidepressant that never really got off the ground. For one thing, it is only available in a single dose: 90 mg/week. That's supposed to be equivalent to 20 mg/day, but there are enough pharmacokinetic variations in this weekly tablet to doubt that. At steady state, the weekly version only achieves half the average concentration of the daily pill. The troughs are 76% lower and the peaks 170% higher. And then there's the matter of remembering to take a dose on the same day every week. We could go on, but that's probably enough said.

VERDICT

Weekly fluoxetine is a risky venture.

Anticonvulsants and Mood Stabilizers

Instant-release anticonvulsants pose a clear and present danger in epilepsy, where a drop in serum levels can cause breakthrough seizures. That's why most anticonvulsants are available in modified-release form. Things are different in bipolar disorder, where the mood-stabilizing effects of anticonvulsants build slowly and are less vulnerable to serum level fluctuations. MR formulations are not necessary to prevent mood episodes, but they can reduce some side effects by smoothing out the peaks and troughs. In particular, nausea, dizziness, double vision, and tremor improve when those peaks are smoothed out.

Lithium

Most patients prefer MR lithium over IR, and for good reason. The MR cuts the rate of many side effects in half, including nausea, tremor, and possibly cognitive dulling and urinary frequency. One side effect is lower with the IR, though: diarrhea.

There are two MR versions of lithium: lithium ER (Lithobid) and lithium CR (Eskalith). These two have slightly different pharmacokinetics—lithium CR releases slower and has a smoother peak than lithium ER. Some patients appreciate the CR's higher dose (450 mg instead of the ER's 300 mg), as it means they have fewer pills to take.

Both MR versions release lithium more gradually than the IR, a fact appreciated by the stomach (less nausea) and the kidneys. Renal toxicity on lithium is linked to serum levels, and there is some evidence that kidney damage can be avoided by keeping the level below 0.9 mmol/mL. In theory, the MR formulations reduce that risk by smoothing over those peaks.

Another way to reduce lithium's renal risks is to give the entire dose at night. That strategy worked better than twice-a-day dosing in a few controlled studies, and it makes sense with lithium's half-life of 18–24 hours (Girardi P et al, *Drugs R D* 2016;16(4):293–302). But wait. Didn't we just say that the kidneys do better when lithium's levels are spread out with an MR formulation? The kidneys are finicky organs. They like their lithium levels low, and they also like to get a break from lithium for part of each day. Evening dosing with an MR formulation satisfies both ends.

VERDICT

MR lithium is more tolerable than IR, unless diarrhea is the problem. To protect the kidneys, give lithium all at night and avoid toxic levels.

Valproic Acid

This anticonvulsant has a confusing array of names, but there are really only three versions:

1. Valproic acid or valproate (Depakene). The basic, irreducible molecule is valproic acid, also known as valproate, and the brand name of this is "Depakene," not Depakote.
2. Sodium divalproex (Depakote DR). Sodium divalproex is formed by adding sodium hydroxide to two valproic acid molecules, yielding a molecule that is double the size of valproic acid but that gets cleaved apart in the GI tract, releasing the original single valproic acid. The "kote" in Depakote refers to the fact that it comes in an enteric-coated ("koted") tablet. Depakote tends to cause fewer GI side effects than Depakene, is absorbed more slowly, and has a somewhat longer half-life (12 hours vs 8 hours). Because of the delayed absorption, Depakote is often referred to as "Depakote DR," mostly to distinguish it from its more modern cousin, "Depakote ER."

   Sodium divalproex also comes as a capsule that can be opened up and sprinkled on food, but those "sprinkles" only come as 125 mg, which means your patient would have to open up 10–20 capsules a day to achieve the typical dose.
3. Sodium divalproex extended release (Depakote ER). This is an extended-release version of Depakote DR and is FDA approved for once-daily dosing. In comparative studies, Depakote ER was better tolerated than standard Depakote DR with half as many GI side effects and lower rates of both tremor and weight gain (Smith MC et al, *Epilepsy Behav* 2004;5(5):746–751).

By the way, when you switch a patient to Depakote ER, you have to increase the dose. Why? Because Depakote ER does not fully dissolve until it reaches the colon, and since the colon is not as specialized for absorbing molecules as the small intestine, some of the drug is excreted unchanged. In practice, this means that in order to make up for the unabsorbed portion, you have to dose the medication 10%–20% higher than the dose a patient would receive with Depakote IR or DR.

You'll also need to finesse the timing when checking serum levels on Depakote ER. Serum levels are checked at the trough, or lowest level of the drug. With Depakote ER, that is 21–24 hours after the last dose, but with other versions the trough is about 12 hours. So if your patient takes their dose in the evening, they'd need to get their level drawn just before the labs close at 5 pm the next day. However, if they do get it drawn in the morning, you can estimate the true trough level by multiplying the morning level by 0.75 (Damegunta SR, *Indian J Psychol Med* 2014;36(3):349–350).

TABLE 5-5. Three Versions of Valproic Acid

Generic Name	Brands and Synonyms	U.S. Release	Dosing
Valproic acid	Valproate, Depakene	1978	BID–TID
Sodium divalproex	Divalproex EC, Depakote DR, Depakote Sprinkles	1983	BID
Divalproex ER	Depakote SA	2002	QD

VERDICT

Depakote ER is preferred for its simpler dosing and more favorable side effect profile. There is little reason to go old-school with valproic acid.

Carbamazepine

There are three versions of carbamazepine:

1. Carbamazepine IR (Tegretol) is the basic molecule. It has a short half-life (10–20 hours) and is typically dosed twice a day in psychiatry. In epilepsy, where irregular serum levels are much more risky, it is dosed three or four times a day.
2. Carbamazepine ER (Carbatrol, Equetro) is a capsule filled with a combination of immediate- and extended-release beads. Equetro is FDA approved in bipolar disorder, but as of this writing, it's also the only version of carbamazepine that is not available as a generic. Carbatrol (approved for epilepsy) is identical to Equetro, however, and can be prescribed as a generic (as carbamazepine ER).
3. Carbamazepine XR (Tegretol XR) is an OROS tablet that uses an osmotic pump similar to Concerta. Its pharmacokinetics are similar to those of the beaded carbamazepine ER, but the XR has slightly more variability between the peaks and troughs (20% vs 12%).

Both MR versions are better tolerated than IR carbamazepine, with lower rates of dizziness, double vision, fatigue, and imbalance (Powell G et al, *Cochrane Database Syst Rev* 2010;(1):CD007124). Low doses of carbamazepine MR can be given all at night (eg, below 800 mg). Beyond that, tolerability usually improves with BID dosing, but most patients prefer a smaller dose in the morning and a larger portion in the evening to minimize sedation.

VERDICT

Start most patients on carbamazepine ER. It's a generic equivalent to the version that's FDA approved in bipolar, is better tolerated than the IR, and has slightly better pharmacokinetics than the XR.

Lamotrigine

Lamotrigine is available in several formulations: XR, orally disintegrating tablets (ODT), and chewable tablets. All are available as generics.

The XR version was designed to improve adherence in epilepsy, where lamotrigine is usually dosed twice a day. However, lamotrigine's half-life is a solid 24 hours, so that kind of conservative dosing is only necessary in epilepsy, where a minor slip in serum levels could spell disaster. The XR formulation does improve on a few side effects, specifically dizziness, imbalance, and nausea, which is the main reason to consider it in psychiatry (Ramey P et al, *Epilepsy Res* 2014;108(9):1637–1641). On the other hand, its extended duration may be an impediment to patients who have insomnia or vivid dreams on the drug.

For those who have difficulty swallowing, the cherry- or peppermint-flavored ODT version is a good choice. Psychiatric patients preferred lamotrigine ODT for its ease of swallowing in a comparative study from the aptly titled *Journal of Patient Preference and Adherence* (Sajatovic M et al, *Patient Prefer Adherence* 2013;7:411–417).

Lamotrigine chewable tablets (which can also be dissolved in water) are not generally used in psychiatry. They are useful for young children with epilepsy and only come in small doses (5 and 25 mg).

VERDICT

Lamotrigine XR is preferred for patients with dizziness, imbalance, or nausea on the drug, and the ODT version will be favored by patients who don't like the bitter taste of the pill.

Antipsychotics

Quetiapine (Seroquel) and paliperidone (Invega) are the only antipsychotics that are available as MRs. Paliperidone was originally released as an MR, and no IR versions are available. That might seem like an odd choice, given that the IR version already has a 23-hour half-life, but the MR formulation improved paliperidone's tolerability, allowing patients to start the antipsychotic at a clinically effective dose without the need for titration (Chue PS et al, *Expert Rev Neurother* 2012;12(12):1399–1410).

Quetiapine

First introduced in 2007, quetiapine XR allows once-daily dosing for this antipsychotic that was traditionally dosed twice a day. This is particularly useful in schizophrenia, mania, and mixed states, where doses beyond 300 mg per day are usually needed. Those higher doses can cause hypotension and falls as the serum level peaks, and the XR reduces that risk by smoothing out the serum levels.

On the other hand, the XR formulation can linger too long, causing daytime sedation. This problem is partially overcome by dosing it 4–5 hours before bed, which is about how long it takes for the level, and hence the sedation, to peak (by contrast, the IR version peaks in about 2 hours). Taking the XR earlier in the evening makes it less likely to cause fatigue the next morning. However, keep in mind that the dose needs to be spaced out an hour away from a meal because food causes the XR mechanism to break down, releasing the entire dose at once.

VERDICT

At doses below 400 mg, use IR quetiapine and dose it all at night. Use the XR version if higher doses are required or the patient is prone to orthostasis.

Stimulants

For an extended-release enthusiast, the world of psychostimulants is Jerusalem and Mecca combined. It's where extended-release formulations all began, and from where dozens have been devised and marketed over the years. Due to this embarrassment of riches, this section will be fairly long—but we hope that it will give you the tools you need to sort through all the stimulant options as you decide on which to offer your patients.

There are two basic types of stimulants: methylphenidate (Ritalin and its knockoffs) and amphetamine (Adderall, Dexedrine, Vyvanse, & company). Within each of these broad categories are subcategories with different mixtures of the drug's isomers. To understand these variations, you have to understand something about isomers.

Isomers are mirror-image molecules of one another, and each stimulant comes in two isomer forms. Although they look alike, they don't work the same way in the brain, just as right-handed scissors don't work well for left-handed people.

The methylphenidate isomers are dex- and levo-methylphenidate. Methylphenidate products are either a 1:1 mix of these two (eg, Ritalin, Concerta, and others labeled "methylphenidate"), or 100% pure dexmethylphenidate (eg, Focalin). There are no pure levo- products because this isomer has little CNS activity.

The main amphetamine isomers are dextro- and levo-amphetamine. Of the two, dextroamphetamine is more potent, with a higher abuse potential and greater appetite suppressant effects. Levoamphetamine is longer lasting and causes more cardiac side effects. Amphetamines are available as a 3:1 dextro:levo mixture (mixed amphetamine salts, eg, Adderall), as a 1:1 mix (Evekeo), and as pure dextroamphetamine (Dexedrine and, in prodrug form, Vyvanse).

Next we'll look at how these basic products are wrapped in various drug-delivery packages.

The Methylphenidates

With an onset of 15–30 minutes and a duration of 3–5 hours, methylphenidate IR is quick to act and quick to fade away. A series of formulations have appeared to extend its effects, beginning with wax-coated tablets in 1987 (eg, Ritalin SR and Metadate ER). These were supposed to release equal doses of methylphenidate 4 hours apart, but they often got the timing wrong by an hour or two, so they've fallen out of use. The one advantage of wax tablets is their low cost, but wax capsules (eg, Metadate CD) work better for a similar price.

The next generation of methylphenidate MRs started hitting the market in 2000. Most of these are mixtures of immediate- and extended-release beads that cause two biphasic peaks in their serum levels. Concerta stands out for its single, monophasic peak, made possible by an osmotic delivery that gradually releases the drug. Concerta is favored for its long, 12-hour duration and generic price point, but its slow speed of onset can be a drawback. It takes 1–2 hours for Concerta to start working, which can be a problem for patients trying to get to school or work on time.

That problem could be fixed with a small dose of methylphenidate IR in the morning, but several brands have also stepped in with their own solutions. First came Ritalin LA, which is packed with 50% immediate-release

TABLE 5-6. Methylphenidate Formulations

Brand	Mechanism	Duration (hr)	Release Date
Ritalin, Methylin chew tabs, liquid	IR	3–5	1955
Ritalin SR, Methylin ER, Metadate ER	Wax coating	4–8	1987
Ritalin LA	Mixed beads	6–9	2000
Metadate CD	Mixed beads	8–10	2001
Aptensio XR*	Mixed beads	12	2015
Adhansia XR*	Mixed beads	16	2019
Concerta	Osmotic extended release (ER)	12	2000
QuilliChew ER*	Ion exchange resin	8	2015
Quillivant XR liquid*	Liquid XR	12	2012
Cotempla XR-ODT*	Ion exchange resin	12	2017
Daytrana patch*	Transdermal patch	12	2006
Jornay PM*	Delayed release	8–11	2018

*Available as brand only

and 50% XR beads for patients who need more effect in the first 4 hours after taking it. However, Ritalin LA peters out 3–6 hours before Concerta does. Another beaded system, Aptensio XR, attempts to balance both ends with XR beads that last longer than Ritalin LA's. The result is an onset that's 2–3 times faster than Concerta's and a 12-hour duration that's nearly identical. Those specs might make Aptensio XR the preferred choice for many patients if cost was not an issue.

A novel solution to the morning problem is to take the stimulant at night and have it turn on in the morning through a long delayed-release mechanism. Jornay PM, which takes effect 8–10 hours after ingestion, was the first to try this approach, and others are under development.

The remaining methylphenidate MRs stand out more for their ease of swallowing than their duration of action. Those include liquid (Quillivant), chewable (QuilliChew), and orally disintegrating (Cotempla XR-ODT). All are clinically sound but financially costly. Another alternative is the Daytrana patch, but it has significant drawbacks. The patch was developed to allow easy on-off effects, but it is slow to start (1–2 hours) and lingers for 2–3 hours, or even up to 5 hours in some patients, after its removal. It is prone to falling off, and can lead to mild overdoses with excess heat. It can also cause *leukoderma*, or permanent loss of skin pigmentation around the application site. The amphetamine varieties have yet to appear as a patch, but one is under development from Noven Pharmaceuticals.

Dexmethylphenidate

The dexmethylphenidate stimulants once went by the brand name Focalin, but both are generic now. Although they isolate the more potent dex- isomer, there is little evidence that they are any better than methylphenidate as long as the doses are comparable. Methylphenidate 20 mg = dexmethylphenidate 10 mg; the dose is cut in half to adjust for the dex- isomer's higher potency. Dexmethylphenidate is rumored to cause less insomnia and appetite suppression than methylphenidate, but head-to-head studies to prove that claim are lacking.

TABLE 5-7. Dexmethylphenidate Formulations

Brand	Mechanism	Duration (hr)	Release Date
Dexmethylphenidate (Focalin)	IR	3–5	2001
Dexmethylphenidate XR (Focalin XR)	Mixed beads	8–12	2005

The Amphetamines

Released in 1935, amphetamine is the original stimulant. Throughout its long career, the drug has sometimes fallen out of favor, only to return in a new formulation. The original brand of racemic amphetamine, Benzedrine, was tarnished in the 1960s by a highly publicized epidemic of Benzedrine ("bennies") abuse. It continued as dextroamphetamine (Dexedrine), even though this potent isomer has an abuse potential that rivals that of Benzedrine. The mix of amphetamine salts we know as Adderall was originally marketed for obesity as Oleptro. The name was changed to Adderall (as in "ADD for All") in the 1990s after physicians became concerned about the risk-benefit ratio of amphetamines in weight control. In the last decade, racemic amphetamine was reintroduced as Evekeo, even though it is identical to the Benzedrine of 1935.

That leaves us with three basic mixtures of amphetamine: racemic (1:1 dextro:levo), mixed salts (3:1 dextro:levo), and pure, 100% dextroamphetamine. Once you settle on the mixture that is best suited for your patient, the next step is to figure out which formulation they need. Racemic amphetamine (Evekeo) lasts a generous 9 hours and is not available in MR form. The other amphetamines last 4–6 hours and have several MRs available that extend that duration to 10–16 hours (Table 5-9).

Besides extending the duration, MR stimulants also reduce the abuse potential. Lisdexamfetamine (Vyvanse) takes this one step further by locking down the dextroamphetamine molecule with a lysine bond, preventing the drug from becoming active until the lysine is cleaved off in the bloodstream. This interesting formulation accomplishes two things. First, it slows down the drug's release, and second, it makes Vyvanse impossible to abuse by snorting—though it can still be abused by swallowing.

Compared to other versions of dextroamphetamine, Vyvanse's metabolism is more steady and consistent, which translates to a longer duration of action and smoother effects throughout the day (Mattingly GW et al, *Postgrad Med* 2017;129(7):657–666). Those advantages make Vyvanse the preferred form of pure dextroamphetamine in all respects except cost. The dextro- isomer also has unique anorexic effects, which led Vyvanse to gain FDA approval in binge-eating disorder in the higher dose range (50–70 mg).

TABLE 5-8. Racemic Amphetamine (1:1 dextro:levo)

Brand	Mechanism	Duration (hr)	Release Date
Evekeo, Evekeo ODT	IR	9	1935

TABLE 5-9. Mixed Amphetamine Salts (3:1 dextro:levo)

Brand	Mechanism	Duration (hr)	Release Date
Adderall	IR	4–6	1996
Adderall XR	Mixed beads	10–12	2001
Adzenys XR-ODT and ER-liquid	Ion exchange resin	10–12	2016–2017
Dyanavel XR liquid	Ion exchange resin	12	2016
Mydayis	Mixed beads	16	2017

TABLE 5-10. Dextroamphetamine (100% dextro)

Brand	Mechanism	Duration (hr)	Release Date
Dexedrine, Zenzedi	IR	4–6	1937
Dextroamphetamine ER (Spansules)	Mixed beads	6–10	1952
Vyvanse	Prodrug	9–14	2007

Methamphetamine

There is one more stimulant that we left off the list: methamphetamine (Desoxyn). You'll need to know about it if only to avoid it. This structural analogue of amphetamine was popular as a diet pill and ADHD treatment from the 1940s until the 1960s. While there are occasional patients who seem to be particularly responsive to methamphetamine, its neurotoxicity and high addictive potential make it unsuitable for most if not all patients (Kim B et al, *Biomol Ther (Seoul)* 2020;28(5):381–388).

CHAPTER 6

Transdermal and Intranasal Delivery

ORAL DELIVERY OF MEDICATIONS is the standard, but we've learned that the process of GI absorption can take a big bite out of a drug's bio-availability. Both transdermal and intranasal administration largely bypass first-pass metabolism in the liver, ensuring faster and more reliable drug delivery and avoiding GI irritation. Once in the bloodstream, transdermal and intranasal medications still pass through the liver, but only a small portion (around 10%) of the medication makes it there—meaning that there are fewer drug metabolites around to cause mischief.

Transdermal Medications in Psychiatry

Transdermal Selegiline Patch (EMSAM)

The MAOI antidepressant EMSAM (transdermal selegiline) was the first major psychiatric medication to be released as a patch, and it was for a good reason. Standard MAOIs can cause a hypertensive crisis when people ingest tyramine-rich foods like aged cheese. Usually, when we ingest tyramine, it is broken down by the enzyme monoamine oxidase. But if you have an MAOI on board, you are inhibiting the MAO enzyme and therefore caus-ing a buildup of tyramine. Tyramine is an amino acid, and one of its actions in the body is to cause the release of catecholamines from nerve terminals. Catecholamines include epinephrine and norepinephrine, both of which can cause hypertension, and MAOIs can cause dangerously high blood pressure when taken with tyramine-rich foods.

How does EMSAM minimize this problem? Since it is absorbed trans-dermally, it mostly bypasses the GI tract and therefore does not signifi-cantly inhibit the MAO enzymes there. This allows ingested tyramine to be metabolized normally so it doesn't build up to dangerous levels.

Unfortunately, this is not a major triumph for EMSAM because only the lowest dose (6 mg/day) is completely free of these food interactions. Higher doses will inhibit tyramine's breakdown, which is a problem because EMSAM's antidepressant effects are dose dependent. Most patients eventually need up to 9–12 mg, at which point dietary restrictions around tyramine become necessary. It's also not clear that EMSAM works as well as the other MAOIs that, unlike EMSAM, have been shown to work in treatment-resistant depression.

While EMSAM doesn't completely get around the food restriction, its transdermal delivery does make it more tolerable than traditional MAOIs. The patch has few side effects outside of skin irritation.

VERDICT

MAOIs are preferred in atypical depression (overeating, oversleeping, heavy feelings in limbs), and EMSAM's tolerability makes it a good option there. However, it isn't known to work in treatment-resistant depression, and its transdermal delivery only gets around the food limitations in the lower dose range.

Transdermal Asenapine (Secuado)

Secuado is a transdermal form of the atypical antipsychotic asenapine (Saphris). It was released in 2019, which was a year before Saphris' patent expired. Like Saphris, Secuado is FDA approved in schizophrenia, but unlike Saphris it lacks approval in bipolar disorder.

The main difference between Saphris and Secuado is in their pharmaco-kinetics. Saphris is administered under the tongue and is absorbed directly through the oral mucosa. Like other sublingual agents, Saphris comes on fast, peaking within an hour. Transdermal asenapine, on the other hand, takes 12–24 hours to peak.

So why would you choose Secuado over Saphris? The only rationales we could find came from industry-sponsored papers, and they don't hold up well to scrutiny:

1. *Unlike Saphris, Secuado does not leave a bad taste (dysgeusia).* True, the original formulation of Saphris had an awful taste. That problem, however, was largely fixed when the manufacturer added a cherry flavor.
2. *Secuado has no food and drink restrictions.* Food and drink do interfere with Saphris' absorption in the oral mucosa, but this is not a major

drawback because they only need to be avoided for 10 minutes after the dose.

3. *Secuado bypasses first-pass metabolism.* This is true, but since Saphris is absorbed through the oral membrane, it largely bypasses the first-pass effect as well.

4. *As a transdermal patch, Secuado improves adherence.* The idea here is that caregivers can visually check to make sure that the patch is on—whereas they can't ensure that a patient has taken an oral medication. While this has theoretical appeal, there is no empirical evidence that Secuado improves adherence over Saphris. Indeed, since Saphris can't be cheeked, or peeled off later like the patch can, it might provide better support when adherence is a struggle.

When it comes to the bottom line—side effects—Secuado looks virtually identical to Saphris except for an additional nuisance: skin irritation, which affected 1 in 7 patients and caused 1 in 200 to stop the medication (Citrome L et al, *J Clin Psychiatry* 2020;82(1):20m13602).

TABLE 6-1. Asenapine: Sublingual Saphris vs Transdermal Secuado

	Saphris	Secuado
Dose conversion	10 mg/day	3.8 mg/day
	15 mg/day	5.7 mg/day
	20 mg/day	7.6 mg/day
Unique side effects	Unpleasant taste	Skin irritation (15%)
Pharmacokinetics	Faster Tmax (1 hr), same half-life (30 hr), same drug interactions	Slower Tmax (12–24 hr)
Advantages	Fatigue can be minimized by taking the entire dose at night	Transdermal patches preferred by some patients and families
Disadvantages	Cannot eat or drink within 10 minutes of taking it	Absorption is decreased by oily, hairy skin, and increased by heat
Monthly cost	$120 and dropping	$1,200

VERDICT

It's hard to see an advantage with transdermal asenapine, and economic factors will point most patients toward the generic, sublingual form.

Other Transdermal Patches Used in Psychiatry

Nicotine Patch

The nicotine patch was released in 1991 as a prescription and transitioned to over-the-counter in 1996 to improve access. Overall, it works as well as other nicotine replacement therapies, but some smokers prefer the faster onset of nicotine gum, vapes, or nasal spray. Combining the two offers the best of both worlds. The long-acting patch lessens cravings overall, while the immediate-release nicotine provides a quick fix for breakthrough cravings. If insomnia is a problem on the patch, it can usually be managed by removing it in the evening. Nicotine patches also have promising studies for depression and age-related cognitive decline.

Methylphenidate Patch (Daytrana)

Daytrana is a methylphenidate patch that is useful for patients who need coverage in the evening hours but also need an "off switch" to halt drug delivery before sleep. See Chapter 5 for our discussion of its advantages and disadvantages.

Clonidine Patch

The alpha-agonist clonidine is available as IR, ER, and a weekly transdermal patch. Although it is applied once a week, the patch produces serum levels that are similar to those of the IR and ER—and even a little steadier. The patch is also better tolerated when it comes to sedation and dry mouth. So what's the catch? Like many patches, it can irritate the skin (Pastore MN et al, *Br J Pharmacol* 2015;172(9):2179–2209). Also, transdermal clonidine lacks FDA approval in psychiatry. Only clonidine ER (Kapvay) holds that status, in ADHD.

Still, the patch has been used successfully in half a dozen psychiatric trials, including trials in ADHD and a few other conditions where clonidine has shown off-label potential: opioid withdrawal, nicotine cessation, tics, autism, and PTSD.

The patch is available in 0.1, 0.2, and 0.3 mg/day doses, which are equivalent to the same mg/day in the IR form. The conversion from ER to transdermal is less exact, as only 70%–90% of the ER form actually gets absorbed (ie, 0.3 mg/day of the ER formulation is equivalent to about 0.21–0.27 mg/day IR).

Rivastigmine Patch (Exelon)

Rivastigmine is an anticholinesterase inhibitor used to treat dementia. Gastrointestinal side effects often limit the oral form, so a transdermal patch was developed in hopes of improving its tolerability by smoothing the peak serum levels. The strategy succeeded. In a large head-to-head trial, 72% of caregivers preferred the patch because it had fewer side effects and was easier to dose (it is dosed once a day, while oral rivastigmine is a twice-a-day med).

Managing Skin Irritation

Skin irritation is a common theme with all these patches, which can cause problems that range from mild irritation to bullous conflagrations. Patients can reduce those risks by avoiding harsh soaps, applying a lipid-rich moisturizer a few hours before putting the patch on, and gently cleaning away any residual adhesive after removing the patch. Rotating the delivery site also helps. If the problem persists, prescribe a steroid ointment (eg, 2.5% hydrocortisone cream) to apply before adhering the patch, or refer to a dermatologist for further guidance.

VERDICT

Keep transdermal clonidine and rivastigmine in your toolbox—both of these patches are an improvement on their tolerability. Nicotine patches are also useful to help smokers reduce cravings. Daytrana, however, is seriously hindered by the risk of permanent skin discoloration.

TABLE 6-2. The Pros and Cons of Transdermal Patches

Pros	Cons
Sustained release at a steady rate with fewer peaks and troughs (as long as the patch stays on)	Slower onset, longer duration
Usually has less variability in absorption compared to oral	Oil, sweat, and hair reduce absorption, while hot temperatures speed it up
Fewer side effects from metabolites and GI irritation	Skin irritation
Drug delivery can be stopped by pulling it off	Patch can fall off accidentally, and the medication still lingers after the patch is removed
Simplifies adherence through once-daily (or, for some, weekly) dosing	Stigma of wearing it

Intranasal Medications in Psychiatry

While transdermal medications are slower to act than oral ones, the nasal route speeds up medications' effects through the rich vascular supply of the nose. Some medications can even get into the CNS directly through the olfactory pathways, bypassing the tight blood-brain barrier.

Esketamine

Ketamine and its enantiomer esketamine have a hard time getting from the GI tract to the brain because they are extensively metabolized in the liver. Only 10%–20% of oral ketamine makes it past the liver. The sublingual route improves on this a little (30% survives liver metabolism), while intranasal and intravenous delivery brings it closer to 100%. Ketamine is usually given intravenously, but the manufacturer of esketamine chose the intranasal route for convenience.

Naloxone

When an opioid overdose shuts off the respiratory system, rapid action makes the difference between life and death. The opioid antagonist naloxone achieves that when given intranasally or intramuscularly, and the intranasal route is the preferred route for home delivery by the patient's caregivers. Some people wonder how this intranasal spray can work in an unconscious person who can't sniff. As a sophisticated psychopharmacologist, you can tell them that the key is for the drug to make contact with the nasal mucosa and its rich blood supply and that no sniffing is required for absorption. Bystanders are instructed to spray into one nostril initially, and can spray additional doses into the other nostril after 2 minutes if there is no response.

Naloxone lasts only 30–60 minutes, so caregivers may need to give multiple doses to keep the patient alive while they await EMS. And—while it may save a life—the patient may not thank their rescuer right away. Naloxone will usually precipitate opioid withdrawal symptoms like restlessness, agitation, nausea, vomiting, a fast heart rate, and sweating.

Since 2020, the FDA has required that physicians discuss naloxone before prescribing opioids and highly recommends this conversation with patients who are at risk for opioid overdose. That includes patients who are often encountered in outpatient psychiatry: those who recreationally use opioids, have a history of opioid overdoses, or are taking a benzodiazepine along with an opioid from another doctor.

Oxytocin

This "bonding" hormone has been used in an intranasal form with varying results to try to improve social connection in autistic adults and children. While trials to date have been small, the approach is promising enough and generally apparently safe enough for reasonable consideration as a possible adjunct treatment (Parker KJ et al, *Proc Natl Acad Sci USA* 2017;114(30):8119–8124).

Aromatherapy: The Original Intranasal Route

Some of your patients may already be using intranasal psychotropics through aromatherapy. Lavender oil has anxiolytic and sleep-inducing effects that may be unrelated to its pleasant scent. Aromatized lavender reduced anxious behavior in mice even when the animals were unable to smell. The bioactive compounds in lavender oil have multiple pharmacodynamic effects, including serotonin-1A agonism, NMDA antagonism, and GABA-ergic properties. An oral extract of lavender, Silexan, is licensed for generalized anxiety disorder in 14 countries and available over-the-counter in the US as CalmAid.

Through the Lungs: Oral Inhalation

Inhaled Loxapine

Like the intranasal route, oral inhalation allows rapid entry and quick effects. We only have one inhaled medication in psychiatry: loxapine inhalation powder (Adasuve). Inhaled alprazolam is under development for epilepsy, but its rapid onset may prove to be a liability as this inhaled benzo is more addictive than the slow-acting oral. The hypnotic zolpidem is available as a sprayable version (Zolpimist), but this is absorbed in the mouth much like a sublingual med and should not be inhaled.

Inhaled loxapine is FDA approved for agitation in bipolar disorder and schizophrenia and is sometimes used off label for agitation in borderline personality disorder. The powder delivery system is similar to other inhaled medications and easy to use. Inhaled loxapine is well tolerated in adults and in children, with sedation and taste changes (dysgeusia) as the most common side effects. The main drawback of inhaled loxapine is that it is contraindicated in respiratory illnesses associated with bronchospasms, including asthma and COPD, and that medical history may be hard to verify in the emergency settings it's used in. Loxapine is not available for outpatient use, and facilities must be registered with a REMS program to use it.

Inhaled loxapine works quickly, peaking in a few minutes and reaching full clinical effect in 10–20 minutes. Its half-life is about 7 hours in adults and 15 hours in children.

Injectable Medications

INJECTIONS ARE GIVEN IN PSYCHIATRY for various reasons:

- Short-acting intramuscular (IM) injections for agitated patients who refuse oral meds
- Long-acting depot injections for patients who, for various reasons, cannot or will not take oral meds consistently
- Intravenous (IV) injections in rare cases, such as when ultrarapid action is needed in medically ill patients with IV access

Short-Acting IM Injections for Agitation

When rapid action is of the essence and you are unable to calmly encourage your patient to try an oral or sublingual medication, go with IM injection. IMs generally produce an effect within 5 minutes, four times faster than most oral meds. The reason they are so rapid is that the medication is injected deep within the muscles, which are richly supplied with blood vessels, and these vessels bypass portal circulation and go directly to the brain.

However, there are some oral formulations with speeds that rival IM meds. One small study of 42 patients found that orally disintegrating Zyprexa Zydis and risperidone liquid worked just as quickly as IM haloperidol for agitated psychotic patients (Hsu WY et al, *J Clin Psychopharmacol* 2010;30(3):230–234).

One thing most clinicians don't realize is that IM injections are actually not that reliable, and that they have a relatively high "failure rate." An IM "failure" refers to situations where the needle does not reach far enough to actually penetrate the muscle, and instead is injected into the subcutaneous tissue. There's much less vasculature in the subcutaneous tissue, so absorption is likely to be poorer and less drug will be delivered to the brain. The failure rate ranges from 50% to 70% and is higher in patients with thicker subcutaneous tissue, including women and people who are obese (Soliman E et al, *Biodes Manuf* 2018;1(3):161–170).

Is there anything you can do to improve the chances that your patient's IM injection will be successful? Though you are unlikely to actually give the injection, you can encourage the nurses you work with to follow these guidelines:

- Choose ventrogluteal over dorsogluteal sites. Gluteal injections can be given in two areas. The dorsogluteal area is the easiest to locate (it's in the upper-left quadrant of the buttocks), doesn't require as much training, and is easier to access when you are dealing with a highly agitated patient. However, the ventrogluteal site (in the hip, just below the femur) has a higher success rate because there is less subcutaneous tissue.

- Use the Z-track method. With the non-injecting hand, you laterally displace the skin and the subcutaneous tissue prior to injection. This enhances the likelihood that the needle will reach the IM area.

- Use the right needle size. Needles used for IM injections are typically 25–38 mm (1–1.5 in) long and 19–22 gauge. Needle gauge is the measure of the thickness of the needle and ranges from 7 gauge (the largest) to 33 (the smallest) on the Stubs scale. 21-gauge needles are most commonly used for IM injections. The person giving the injection will usually choose a needle based on the size of the patient—longer needles are needed for more obese patients. However, in the case of long-acting injectables, the dose pack usually comes with a needle that the manufacturers require for the injection, which ensures that the right needle is chosen for the given patient.

The bottom line is that, in an emergency situation with an acutely agitated patient, the IM injection is not the panacea that we often assume. If your patient is obese, the medication may not be well absorbed—so don't be surprised if the injection doesn't seem to have much effect. For such patients, consider choosing an orally disintegrating or liquid version.

Let's go through some of the more common short-acting IM medications that we use in psychiatry, primarily for treating agitation. In a later section, we'll take a close look at the long-acting injectables.

Short-Acting IM Antipsychotics

Haloperidol (Haldol) and the Haloperidol Cocktails

IM haloperidol is still the gold standard for rapid tranquilization because it has a long track record, and no other drug has ever been shown to be more effective—and indeed there have been many such comparative studies. The problem with haloperidol is that it has a high rate of dystonia when used alone—as high as 50%. That is why IM haloperidol is usually given with two other drugs as follows: haloperidol 5–10 mg/lorazepam 1–2 mg/ diphenhydramine 50 mg (or benztropine 1–2 mg)—given either IM or orally. The rationale is that lorazepam reduces agitation and diphenhydramine prevents dystonia and extrapyramidal side effects (EPS), but recent research indicates that lorazepam alone may be sufficient to prevent EPS (Bak M et al, *Eur Psychiatry* 2019;57:78–100). An advantage of using haloperidol + lorazepam alone is that these meds can be administered in one syringe. When diphenhydramine or benztropine are mixed with haloperidol, a precipitate forms within minutes, leading most hospital pharmacies to recommend separate syringes.

Olanzapine (Zyprexa)

Many inpatient psychiatrists are finding good success by choosing IM olanzapine over haloperidol combinations. A four-way comparison of IM agents found that olanzapine was just as effective as the haloperidol/ midazolam combination, and that both options were more effective than either ziprasidone or haloperidol plus promethazine (Mantovani C et al, *J Clin Psychopharmacol* 2013;33(3):306–312).

Olanzapine + Benzos—Safe or Unsafe?

For patients who don't respond to IM olanzapine, you may be tempted to add IM lorazepam or another benzodiazepine. If you prescribe this duo, you will likely get a call from the hospital pharmacist informing you that the combination is too dangerous. This is based on a 2005 warning issued by Eli Lilly (olanzapine's manufacturer) about 29 post-marketing fatalities linked to IM olanzapine/IM benzodiazepine combinations from January 2004 to September 2005. However, a closer examination of the data has raised questions about whether any of the deaths were actually causally related to the combination, and a recent review concluded that the combination is likely safe (Williams AM, *Ment Health Clin* 2018;8(5):208–213).

Ziprasidone (Geodon)

IM ziprasidone has gained popularity in some hospitals because it appears to quell agitation without the sedative effects of haloperidol and olanzapine. However, studies show that it's overall less effective than IM olanzapine or IM haloperidol/benzo combination (Mantovani C et al, *J Clin Psychopharmacol* 2013;33(3):306–312). While we are often alert to the concern that ziprasidone increases the risk of QTc prolongation, IM haloperidol has the same risk, and this increase in QTc has not translated into an elevated rate of cardiac arrhythmias with ziprasidone.

Aripiprazole (Abilify)

Aripiprazole is no longer available in the short-acting IM version as it was withdrawn by the manufacturer due to poor sales. Its drawbacks included a high risk of akathisia and a low rate of efficacy compared to other second-generation antipsychotic IMs (Wilson MP et al, *West J Emerg Med* 2012;13:26–34).

Chlorpromazine (Thorazine)

Chlorpromazine, the first antipsychotic to be developed, has a long track record of use for agitation, especially in its IM form. This medication's main advantage is a low risk of EPS. Its drawbacks include QTc prolongation, orthostatic dizziness, and a lowered seizure threshold. While these side effects lead some authorities to discourage its use, in the real world of inpatient psychiatry we find that many of our agitated patients respond better to chlorpromazine than any other agent.

IM Benzodiazepines and Anticholinergics

There are three benzodiazepines that can be given IM or IV: lorazepam (Ativan), diazepam (Valium), and midazolam (Versed). Of these three, lorazepam is by far the most popular in psychiatry. It's preferred over diazepam for two reasons: a shorter half-life and a lack of active metabolites. In addition, diazepam's IM absorption tends to be more erratic than

TABLE 7-1. IM Medications Commonly Used for Acute Agitation

	Medication	Dose	Notes
Antipsychotics	Haloperidol	2–10 mg IM every 4–8 hours	Gold standard; should administer with a benzodiazepine or an anticholinergic to prevent dystonia
	Olanzapine	2.5–10 mg IM, max 30 mg/day	Good option as a stand-alone; usage with IM benzos likely safe despite 2005 warning
	Ziprasidone	20–40 mg IM/day	Less sedating but less effective than other agents
	Chlorpromazine	25–50 mg IM, max 200 mg/day	Very sedating and low risk of EPS; drawbacks include orthostasis and—rarely—seizures or QTc prolongation
Benzos	Lorazepam	0.5–2 mg every 4–6 hours, max 10 mg/day	Useful for catatonia, akathisia, and neuroleptic malignant syndrome
	Diazepam	5–10 mg every 3–4 hours	Erratic IM absorption makes it less reliable; mainly used IV for seizures
	Midazolam	5–15 mg IM for acute agitation	Use is limited by respiratory depression
Anticholinergics	Benztropine	1–4 mg IM up to BID	For akathisia or acute dystonia; may be given to prevent EPS
	Diphenhydramine	25–50 mg IM every 4–6 hours	Used for acute dystonia, a disulfiram reaction, or allergic reactions; often given with haloperidol to prevent EPS
	Promethazine	25–50 mg IM every 4–6 hours	Less used in the US in psychiatry

lorazepam's IM absorption. Parenteral diazepam is more commonly used in its IV form for status epilepticus.

What about midazolam? Midazolam is a very short-acting benzodiazepine with a half-life of 1–2 hours, and it has an unusually rapid onset of action. This benzodiazepine is often used in anesthesia before a surgery or colonoscopy because of its rapid onset and strong amnestic effects. Patients typically will not recall anything during the procedure after they receive the injection.

Why isn't midazolam used more often in psychiatry? It's not completely clear, since there were a few studies showing that it's quite effective for agitation. For example, one study in Brazil randomly assigned 301 aggressive or agitated psychotic patients to either 7.5–15 mg IM midazolam or 5–10 mg IM haloperidol/promethazine combination (promethazine is a sedating antihistamine/anticholinergic, similar to Benadryl). Midazolam worked faster than haloperidol—89% of patients given midazolam were tranquil or asleep after 20 minutes compared with 67% of those given the haloperidol combination, a statistically significant difference (TREC Collaborative Group, *BMJ* 2003;327(7417):708–713). One patient on midazolam developed significant respiratory depression—and this may clue us in to why psychiatrists are not using midazolam. It has a reputation of being more likely to cause respiratory depression and profound sedation, though to our knowledge there are no studies comparing it on these variables with other benzodiazepines.

Finally, there are three anticholinergics available in injectable form: diphenhydramine (Benadryl), benztropine (Cogentin), and promethazine (Phenergan). They all have similar onsets of action (around 15 minutes) when given IM. Of the three, diphenhydramine is the most commonly used in the US for the acute treatment of agitation or dystonia.

Long-Acting Injectable Antipsychotics (LAIs)

LAIs can be helpful for patients who are unable to comply with regular oral medication over the long course of these illnesses. Also known as depot medications, LAIs can reduce rates of rehospitalization by 29% in real-world settings compared to treatment with oral antipsychotics (Kim HO et al, *Ann Gen Psychiatry* 2020;19:1). Another advantage of LAIs is that the average peak dose is 20%–30% lower than orals, which means that side effects tend to be more manageable. Moreover, patients may be stable for up to a week after a missed dose, giving you more time to see them before they decompensate.

We will go through each of the currently available LAI antipsychotics below. For each one we'll cover the following aspects, which will be helpful as you consider which to choose for your patients:

- *Mechanism of release.* Release mechanisms are constantly evolving, and it's helpful to have a basic understanding of the underlying biomechanics because they affect important parameters such as onset of action and pain at the injection site.

- *Pharmacokinetics.* You'll need to know the Tmax to make accurate dosing decisions.
- *Oral overlap.* Agents differ on how quickly you can titrate up the dose. This is important because antipsychotics that require gradual titration will need to be started through the oral route before transitioning to LAI. This process is called the "oral overlap," and it has two disadvantages. First, it makes the process of dosing a bit more complex, which admittedly is not a huge deal. Second, if the patient is refusing to take oral meds (but accepting an injection, either under court order or voluntarily), you'll have to choose a different LAI or risk a decompensation while waiting for levels to become therapeutic.
- *Dosing.* We'll specify the dosing intervals and describe how to convert from a standard oral dose to the appropriate injectable dose.

Haloperidol Decanoate

Mechanism of release: Haloperidol is combined with decanoic acid (a long-chain fatty acid) in an esterification reaction to create Haldol decanoate, which is dissolved in sesame oil and injected. The oil remains in the muscle and the molecule is gradually hydrolyzed, releasing haloperidol into the bloodstream over the course of weeks.

Pharmacokinetics: The plasma concentration of haloperidol gradually rises, and peaks at about 6 days after the injection, falling thereafter. The half-life is about 3 weeks. Steady-state concentration is achieved in 2–4 months.

Oral overlap: Because the Tmax occurs about a week after the injection, you need to continue oral haloperidol for at least a week, often for 2–3 weeks to be on the safe side. If your patient does not want to take oral haloperidol, you can eliminate the need for overlap by using the "loading dose" method (20 times oral dose, followed by 10–15 times oral dose in subsequent months).

Dosing: Dosing interval is 4 weeks. For a simple oral to IM conversion, 10–15 times the oral dose will provide you with an effective monthly injection dose. You might think you would need 30 times the oral dose for an equivalent effect spaced over a month, but clinical trials have shown that this lower decanoate dose is indeed as effective as the corresponding oral dose (McEvoy JP, *J Clin Psychiatry* 2006;67(suppl 5):15–18; Haloperidol decanoate [package insert]. Titusville, NJ: Ortho-McNeil Neurologics; 2004).

Prolixin Decanoate (Fluphenazine)

Mechanism of release: Identical to haloperidol decanoate. Fluphenazine is combined with decanoic acid to create a stable esterified compound, which is dissolved in sesame oil and injected. The oil remains in the muscle and the molecule is gradually hydrolyzed, releasing fluphenazine into the bloodstream over the course of weeks.

Pharmacokinetics: There is an early high peak during the first day, and then the concentration declines, with an apparent half-life ranging from 6.8 to 9.6 days following a single injection. The time to reach steady-state concentration is 4–6 weeks.

Oral overlap: Since the concentration peaks quickly, only a 2–3 day oral overlap is required.

Dosing: Dosing interval is 2 weeks to begin and then every 2–4 weeks based on clinical needs. For every 10 mg/day of oral fluphenazine, use 12.5 mg of Prolixin decanoate every 3 weeks. The math doesn't seem to add up, but clinical trials show that this seemingly low depot dose is effective (see fluphenazine package insert).

Abilify Maintena (Aripiprazole)

Mechanism of release: Aripiprazole is dissolved into a prolonged-release suspension that is injected.

Pharmacokinetics: Tmax is 5–7 days.

Oral overlap: Continue oral aripiprazole for 14 days. If the patient is on a different antipsychotic, don't switch them to Maintena unless you know they have tolerated aripiprazole in the past. If they have, you can give the injections and continue the therapeutic dose of that antipsychotic for 14 days.

Dosing: Dosing interval is 4 weeks. 400 mg is the starting and continuing dose.

Aristada (Aripiprazole Lauroxil)

Mechanism of release: After it is injected into the muscle, the aripiprazole lauroxil is first hydrolyzed to N-hydroxymethyl aripiprazole, then hydrolyzed again to aripiprazole.

Pharmacokinetics: Tmax occurs at 27 days.

Oral overlap: 3 weeks of oral aripiprazole.

Dosing: 441 and 882 mg 1-month dosing or a 1064 mg 2-month dose.

CHAPTER 7: Injectable Medications **69**

TABLE 7-2. LAI Antipsychotic Medications

LAI Antipsychotic	Dosing	Release Date	Pros and Cons
Abilify Maintena	Monthly	2013	Well tolerated and effective, although requires a 2-week overlap of oral aripiprazole
Aristada (aripiprazole lauroxil)	Every 6–8 weeks	2017	Well tolerated, effective, and long lasting, although meant to be used after a single dose of Aristada Initio
Aristada Initio (aripiprazole lauroxil)	Single dose initiation	2018	Well tolerated and effective, although meant as a one-time use followed by Aristada
Haloperidol decanoate	Every 4 weeks	1982	Simple conversion from oral, but more frequent administration
Invega Sustenna	Every month	2009	Not approved for mania; not tested for bipolar depression; expensive
Invega Trinza	Every 3 months	2015	Longest lasting, but requires 4 months of Invega Sustenna first
Prolixin decanoate (fluphenazine)	Every 2–4 weeks	1972	First in class and an important advance; however, discontinued in 2018 due to single supplier unable to deliver reliably
Risperdal Consta	Every 2 weeks	1993	More research on efficacy, but 3-week oral overlap and then injections every 2 weeks
Zyprexa Relprevv	Every 2–4 weeks	2009	Low rate of EPS, but rare delirium requires 3-hour observation after injection and registration as a prescriber

Aristada Initio (Aripiprazole Lauroxil Nanocrystal Suspension)

Mechanism of release: Aripiprazole lauroxil is also available as a nanocrystal suspension. Like we saw with the earlier Aristada, the prodrug is first hydrolyzed to N-hydroxymethyl aripiprazole, then hydrolyzed again to aripiprazole. For this preparation, however, the smaller particle size makes the particles dissolve faster to reach therapeutic levels more rapidly.

Pharmacokinetics: Reaches "relevant levels" of aripiprazole in 4 days.

Oral overlap: Given with a single dose of 30 mg oral aripiprazole.

Dosing: 675 mg just the one time, then after the Aristada Initio the regular Aristada can be started in the next 1–10 days.

Zyprexa Relprevv (Olanzapine)

Mechanism of release: The nearly insoluble salt form of olanzapine slowly dissolves and enters the circulation.

Pharmacokinetics: Tmax is about 7 days.

Oral overlap: None needed.

Dosing: 150, 210, 300, and 405 mg doses correspond to 10, 15, 20, and 25 mg/day of oral olanzapine respectively, with injections given every 2–4 weeks.

Risperdal Consta (Risperidone)

Mechanism of release: Cellulose-based microspheres dissolve after 3 weeks in the muscle.

Pharmacokinetics: 3 weeks to full release.

Oral overlap: 3 weeks.

Dosing: 12.5, 25, 37.5, or 50 mg every 2 weeks, corresponding to daily oral dosing of 1, 2–3, 3–4, and 4–5 mg.

Invega Sustenna (Paliperidone)

Mechanism of release: After injection, paliperidone palmitate dissolves slowly, is hydrolyzed to paliperidone, and then moves into the circulation.

Pharmacokinetics: Tmax at 13 days.

Oral overlap: None required.

Dosing: First dose 234 mg, 156 mg 1 week later (give or take 4 days), then 117 mg monthly (give or take 7 days), with other dosing options available (39 mg, 78 mg). Conversion from oral paliperidone to Invega Sustenna ranges: 3 mg converts to 39–78 mg; 6 to 117; 9 to 156; 12 to 234 respectively.

Invega Trinza (Paliperidone)

Mechanism of release: After injection, paliperidone palmitate dissolves slowly, is hydrolyzed to paliperidone, and then moves into the circulation.

Pharmacokinetics: Tmax at 30–33 days.

Oral overlap: No oral overlap is required when starting Trinza, but patients must first be on a stable dose of Invega Sustenna (specifically, at least 4 months on Sustenna with no change in the last 2 doses before switching to Trinza).

Dosing: Once every 3 months, with conversion from 78 mg Sustenna to 273 of Trinza; 117 to 410, 156 to 546, and 234 to 819 respectively.

VERDICT

Haloperidol decanoate is the most affordable of the LAIs, but insurance companies are becoming more generous in their coverage of these medications. Among the branded formulations, Invega has a unique advantage, as patients who tolerate the monthly Sustenna version can be switched to the longer-acting Trinza, allowing a generous 3 months between injections. Invega is only approved in schizophrenia and schizoaffective disorders, however, because several of the studies in bipolar mania were negative.

Subcutaneous (SC) Medications

SC medications are injected in the fatty tissue just between skin and muscle. There are fewer blood vessels in the subcutaneous area than there are in the muscles, so medication effects aren't as rapid. SC injections are rarely used in psychiatry, although this may be changing with the recent introduction of an SC antipsychotic—Risperdal Perseris—and bremelanotide (Vyleesi), an SC injection for women with sexual dysfunction.

Risperdal Perseris (Risperidone)

Risperdal Perseris is a once-monthly SC injectable form of risperidone that was approved in 2018 for treatment of schizophrenia.

Mechanism of release: The liquid forms a depot in the subcutaneous tissue that slowly releases the medication.

Pharmacokinetics: For risperidone there are two peaks, one at 4–6 hours while the depot is forming, then another at 10–14 days; however, for the combination of risperidone and the active metabolite 9-hydroxyrisperidone, the first Tmax occurs at 2 days and the second occurs at 7–11 days.

Oral overlap: None needed.

Dosing: Start with 90 mg monthly (equivalent to 3 mg/day of oral risperidone); can increase to 120 mg monthly (equivalent to 4 mg/day oral).

TABLE 7-3. IV Antipsychotic Medications

Medication	IV Dosing
Aripiprazole	1.7 mg/mL solution given in 5.25–15 mg doses, up to 30 mg/day
Haloperidol	2–10 mg up to every 30 minutes, up to 100 mg/day
Olanzapine	2.5–10 mg IV bolus, up to 30 mg/day
Quetiapine	About 200 mg/day
Ziprasidone	10–20 mg, up to 40 mg/day

Bremelanotide (Vyleesi)

Bremelanotide is an SC injection that's FDA approved for female hypoactive sexual desire disorder (HSDD) in premenopausal women. It is an analogue of the alpha-melanocyte-stimulating hormone, which activates melanocortin in the central and peripheral nervous systems. Women self-administer bremelanotide in the abdomen or thigh at least 45 minutes before sex (its half-life is 2.7 hours, but effects can last up to 24 hours). Unfortunately, skin reactions at the injection site are a common side effect (13%), and 1 in 100 develop hyperpigmentation of the skin at the site. That risk increases the longer bremelanotide is used, and half of the time the discoloration becomes permanent.

Intravenous Medications

Intravenous (IV) medications have a long history of use in psychiatry for catatonia, agitation, and delirium. More recently, two medications have entered the field as rapid-acting IV therapies for depression: ketamine and brexanolone.

IV lorazepam is sometimes used to treat catatonia or agitation when we need a more rapid-acting option than either oral or IM. Its onset of action is 1–3 minutes if administered IV vs 15–30 minutes if administered IM.

IV antipsychotics are sometimes used in medical settings to treat delirium, but the research supporting this use is thin. Recently, two meta-analyses concluded that antipsychotics worked no better than a placebo at treating or preventing delirium, and instead brought additional side effects to the picture, particularly cardiac ones like QTc prolongation (Oh ES et al,

Ann Intern Med 2019;171(7):474–484; Nikooie R et al, *Ann Intern Med* 2019;171(7):485–495).

Brexanolone (Zulresso) was released in 2019 as a treatment for postpartum depression (PPD). Its main advantage is its rapid onset of action, as every week of maternal depression takes a measurable toll on the health of the baby. This medication is given as a 60-hour continuous IV infusion. While effective for depression, brexanolone is expensive and has a complex administration process.

CHAPTER 8

Biotransformation and the Liver

BIOTRANSFORMATION REFERS TO THE VARIOUS WAYS that our bodies change drugs before they leave the body. Those changes usually render the drugs inactive, but in some cases they create new compounds that are even more powerful than the parent compounds. *Excretion* and *elimination*, which we cover in detail in Chapter 9, refer to how drugs actually leave the body—the vast majority of the time, this is via the kidneys or the GI tract. Another term for biotransformation is simply *drug metabolism*, but over time "drug metabolism" has taken on a broader definition encompassing all the things we discuss in this book, including absorption, distribution, biotransformation, and excretion.

Generally, biotransformation involves altering drug molecules to make it easier for them to travel through the kidneys or the intestines. But you should know that some drugs get excreted without being transformed at all. In psychiatry, the most famous of these is lithium, which simply gets diffused into the kidney's tubule system and sent out through the urine. Lithium is known as a metabolically inert drug, although pharmacologically it is highly active and can have quite an effect on the kidney and thyroid, which we discuss in Chapter 9.

Almost all the other drugs that we prescribe, however, undergo various chemical reactions before they can be excreted. There are two primary ways that our bodies alter drugs:

1. Phase I reactions (mostly involving cytochrome P450 enzymes)
2. Phase II reactions, or conjugation (primarily involving glucuronidation)

Phase I Reactions: The P450 System and Others

The enzymes involved in biotransformation have most of their offices in liver cells, specifically in the linings of the sinuous interior membranes called the "smooth endoplasmic reticulum." These enzymes have many names and abbreviations, making some discussions of this topic needlessly confusing. Their official name is "cytochrome P450 enzymes." This is sometimes truncated to "P450 enzymes," and occasionally you'll see the terms "microsomal" or "hepatic" enzymes, which mean the same thing.

The name "cytochrome P450 enzymes" is actually just a bit of researcher jargon. In research laboratories, these enzymes are examined in artificially created spheres of cellular tissue called "microsomal vesicles." When these enzymes are placed in such vesicles, they give off a colored pigment and absorb light at a wavelength of 450 nm. Thus, "cyto" = microsomal vesicles; "chrome" = colored; "P" = pigmented; and "450" = 450 nm wavelength of light.

The P450 enzymes specialize in turning lipophilic ("fat loving") drugs into water-soluble compounds in a process called *Phase I metabolism*. Some medications then undergo a second step where they are joined to another molecule to make them even more water soluble (this is called *Phase II metabolism*; see the next section).

How do drugs become water soluble? By being transformed into "polar" compounds—that is, compounds that are positively charged on one end and negatively charged on the other. These polar molecules are attracted to water, because water is also polar, and the positive side of the drug is attracted to the negative side of H_2O (or in other cases, the negative side of the drug is attracted to the positive side of H_2O). Our kidneys are set up to *excrete* polar compounds and to *reabsorb* lipophilic compounds. If we couldn't polarize things, it would take us months or years to get rid of them. We devote much of Chapter 9 to the kidney in order to torture you into the "wee" hours of the morning.

The P450 enzymes catalyze three major chemical reactions:
- Oxidation: Adding oxygen or removing hydrogen to create a polar molecule
- Reduction: Adding hydrogen or removing oxygen to create a polar molecule
- Hydrolysis: Splitting the molecule and adding a hydrogen atom to one part and a hydroxide group to the other, rendering both new, smaller molecules polar

The point of these reactions is to turn an uncharged molecule into a positively or negatively charged molecule. Once a molecule has a charge (positive or negative), it is more attracted to water (hydrophilic), less attracted to fat (lipophobic), and exits the body more easily.

Oxidation means taking electrons away from a compound, causing it to have a net positive charge. Confusingly, an oxidative reaction does not necessarily mean adding oxygen to the drug. It just means that the drug is left with fewer electrons. There are several ways to achieve this. Fluoxetine, for example, gets oxidized by losing a methyl group (CH_3) and becoming norfluoxetine. (Norfluoxetine happens to be an example of an active metabolite; it continues to block serotonin reuptake transporters until it is further transformed.) Tricyclics get oxidized by gaining a hydroxyl group (OH). Most psych meds are biotransformed through oxidation. Others are biotransformed by *reduction* (adding electrons by adding a hydrogen atom), and still others are biotransformed by *hydrolysis* (adding H_2O, which causes a molecule to split up into two polar molecules). As we saw in Chapter 7, hydrolysis is how the body gradually metabolizes long-acting injectable antipsychotics, such as haloperidol decanoate.

Phase II Reactions: Conjugation

Conjugation means combining a drug with another molecule, called the "conjugating agent." These agents do two things to medications. First, they render them pharmacologically inactive, and second, they make them more water soluble than the original drug and thus less likely to get reabsorbed back into circulation. Conjugating a drug is quite simple conceptually—it's like putting a heavy, weighted suit on a basketball player, rendering them unable to play and causing them to leave the court.

Conjugation is known as "Phase II" because it often occurs after the Phase I reactions in cases where Phase I does not make the drug sufficiently hydrophilic to get eliminated. By far the most common conjugation reaction is *glucuronidation*, in which glucuronic acid ($C_6H_{10}O_6$) is stuck onto a drug, rendering it water soluble (hydrophilic) and lipid insoluble (lipophobic). In psychiatry, lots of drugs are metabolized mainly by glucuronidation, including two mood stabilizers (lamotrigine and valproate) and three benzodiazepines (lorazepam, temazepam, and oxazepam). Glucuronidation is less affected by aging and liver disease than Phase I metabolism, which is why those three benzos are preferred in the elderly.

Glucuronidation is also the site of an important interaction between lamotrigine and valproate. Valproate latches onto the glucuronidation enzyme more aggressively than lamotrigine, shoving lamotrigine aside, which prevents the lamotrigine from being metabolized and thereby increases its levels to about double what they are otherwise. Thus, when a patient is on valproate, you have to start lamotrigine at half the dose (25 mg every other day instead of every day) and titrate in smaller increments than usual.

Let's review the essentials of biotransformation. Your average psychiatric medication gets absorbed through the small intestine, gets distributed by the bloodstream to the liver and then to various organs (especially the brain), and then begins its inexorable journey toward oblivion due to close encounters with various enzymes. These enzymes work hard to turn the drug molecules into polar (hydrophilic) compounds. This involves a variety of maneuvers, including tearing electrons away from the drug (oxidation), stuffing electrons into the drug (reduction), and ripping the molecules apart by offering them some water (hydrolysis). After this "treatment," some drugs are ready to exit right away, either via the kidney or via the bowel. Others require more persuasion and so are conjugated, which generally means being superglued to glucuronic acid, a highly water-soluble compound that effectively ushers drugs out of the body.

Liver Disease and Drug Metabolism

We've reviewed how the liver is supposed to metabolize medications when it is healthy. What happens when our patients present with liver disease? How do we decide if the disease is severe enough to prompt us to change our medication choices or our dosing?

Here are two common scenarios that you should be able to answer by the end of this chapter.

Scenario A: A patient presents to the emergency room for alcohol detox. His labs are normal except for an AST of 110 and an ALT of 60. The ED doc asks you if he should start him on chlordiazepoxide (the standard for your hospital) or oxazepam (the benzodiazepine often used for patients with liver impairment because it lacks active metabolites and is shorter acting). He was going to start oxazepam, but the patient told him that he much prefers chlordiazepoxide because it has worked better for his detoxes in the past. What should you do?

Scenario B: In your outpatient clinic, you have a woman with a history of opioid use disorder who has recently relapsed to fentanyl and wants your help to stop. She says that in the past she has used Vivitrol (monthly naltrexone injection) to help her stay clean. However, over the past year she was diagnosed with chronic hepatitis C, and both her AST and ALT are elevated (about triple the normal values). In the Vivitrol package insert, you read the following: "VIVITROL is contraindicated in: Patients with acute hepatitis or liver failure." What should you do?

Types of Liver Disease Most Common in Psychiatric Practice

Let's start by reviewing the most common causes of liver disease that you are likely to see in your patients. While you are not going to be treating liver disease directly, it's important to know some basics because these different disorders have different implications for your psychotropic prescribing decisions.

Alcoholic Liver Disease

Cause: Direct hepatotoxic effects of excess and chronic alcohol use. Typically starts with asymptomatic mild elevations of transaminases, but eventually can lead to chronic liver disease and alcoholic cirrhosis.

Diagnosis and labs: Excessive drinking plus characteristic labs. In the early stages, AST (SGOT) and ALT (SGPT) may be 2 to 5 times normal, and the AST/ALT ratio is typically 2:1 or more. GGT (gamma-glutamyltransferase) is usually elevated as well and aids in the diagnosis.

Implications for prescribing: Generally, such patients are still able to metabolize drugs in the liver normally, so dosage adjustments are not usually necessary—unless they have cirrhosis (see below).

Drug-Induced Liver Impairment (DILI)

Cause: The vast majority of psychotropic drugs carry warnings in the package insert about the possibility of liver injury, usually based on sporadic case reports. However, most reactions are rare, are characterized by mild elevations of liver enzymes, and are reversible once the drug is discontinued. Furthermore, DILI is not more likely to occur in patients with a history of liver disease.

Diagnosis: DILI is likely to be the culprit in any patient who presents with acute elevation in liver enzymes soon after starting a new medication.

Implications for prescribing: Once the liver recovers, you can prescribe as you normally would, though you should avoid the drug that caused the injury.

Hepatitis B and C

Cause: Both hepatitis B and C begin as acute and can progress to lifelong chronic infections. Of the two, hepatitis C is far more likely to progress to severe liver disease, but on the other hand there are now curative treatments available for it.

Diagnosis: Based on antibody testing and following various hepatic labs over the years.

Implications for prescribing: Unless the patient has progressed to cirrhosis, no dose adjustments are generally needed.

Nonalcoholic Fatty Liver Disease

Cause: The cause is unclear, but it occurs frequently (in about 5% of Americans) and is associated with hyperlipidemia, diabetes, and obesity. There is no specific treatment or cure, but treating the underlying cause or shifting to a healthy diet (eg, Mediterranean) can help.

Diagnosis: Usually presents as mild transaminitis, usually less than 4 times normal values. Usually asymptomatic.

Implications for prescribing: Unless the patient has progressed to cirrhosis, no dose adjustments are generally needed.

Cirrhosis

Cause: The most common causes are alcoholic liver disease, viral hepatitis, and nonalcoholic fatty liver disease. It is the end result of many years of fibrosis and scarring. Liver tissue becomes stiff and impedes the flow of blood, causing pressure to build up in the portal veins. Portal hypertension can then back up into the spleen, causing splenomegaly and the destruction of blood platelets. In addition, portal hypertension can cause other blood vessels to enlarge, causing esophageal varices and gastropathy. Furthermore, the liver cells that usually make albumin and clotting factors become impaired, causing hypoalbuminemia and aggravating clotting problems, which leads to bleeding and easy bruising. Fluid collects in the legs (edema) and in the abdomen (ascites).

Diagnosis: Patients with cirrhosis occasionally are asymptomatic, but as the disease worsens they will present with symptoms such as ascites,

TABLE 8-1. Psychotropic Medication Adjustments in Liver Cirrhosis

No Adjustments Needed	Comment/Rationale
Lithium, gabapentin, topiramate	All three are water soluble and excreted by the kidney with no liver metabolism needed
Temazepam, oxazepam, lorazepam, olanzapine	All are metabolized by Phase II glucuronidation, which is usually preserved in liver disease
Haloperidol	No changes in disposition reported
Baclofen	Only minimal liver metabolism, making it a good choice for the treatment of alcoholism in patients with cirrhosis
Can Be Used With Dosage Adjustments	
Fluoxetine	Lower dose
Escitalopram	Half-life doubled; don't exceed 10 mg
Venlafaxine	Half-life prolonged; reduce dose by 50%
Mirtazapine	Clearance reduced by 30%; reduce dose
Amitriptyline	Increased sedation in cirrhosis; reduce dose
Lamotrigine	Half-life increased; reduce dose in very severe cirrhosis
Carbamazepine	Dose based on CBZ blood levels
Diazepam	Half-life increased 2- to 5-fold; reduce dose
Zolpidem	Half-life increased 2-fold; reduce dose
Drugs to Avoid	
Duloxetine	Half-life increased 3-fold, clearance reduced by 85%
Bupropion	Half-life prolonged; best avoided due to seizure risk
Valproate	Hyperammonemia can worsen encephalopathy
Disulfiram	Risk of hepatic toxicity

edema, jaundice, fatigue, bleeding and easy bruising, and encephalopathy. Lab abnormalities include hyperbilirubinemia, low albumin, and high prothrombin time. Liver enzymes may be normal or only mildly elevated.

Cirrhosis can impede drug metabolism in the following ways:

- Reduced hepatic blood flow can lead to a decreased first-pass effect, causing decreased liver metabolism of drugs and therefore higher serum levels than predicted
- Decreased P450 activity due to hepatic cell injury
- Hypoalbuminemia can lead to less protein binding and therefore higher serum levels of the active free fraction of drugs
- Impaired biliary excretion, causing higher serum levels

Implications for prescribing: Cirrhosis varies in severity, but generally these patients will not be able to clear drugs normally, and you will have to adjust doses of medications that depend on the liver for metabolism. A comprehensive review of medications in cirrhosis was published in 2013 (Lewis JH and Stine JG, *Aliment Pharmacol Ther* 2013;37(12):1132–1156). We've created Table 8-1 based on information from that article.

"Liver Function Tests"—A Misnomer

Most of us consider the main liver function tests to be AST and ALT, but an actual "hepatic panel" consists of several others. In fact, neither AST nor ALT will tell you whether your patient is able to properly metabolize drugs, because neither of them are markers of liver function—instead, they are nonspecific markers of liver injury.

The full panel of hepatic tests can get complicated and the tests are often beyond the scope of what you will be expected to interpret as a psychiatrist, but you should at least be familiar with them.

TABLE 8-2. Common Liver Tests

Nonspecific Markers of Liver Injury	Normal Values
AST	0–40
ALT	0–40
Markers of Biliary Obstruction	
Alkaline phosphatase	40–120
Bilirubin, total	0–1.2
Bilirubin, direct	0–0.4
Markers of Impaired Liver Synthesis	
Protein, total (albumin plus all other proteins)	6–8.5
Albumin	3.5–5.5
Prothrombin time	11–12.5 seconds
Useful for Interpreting Other Labs	
GGT	9–48 units/liter
%CDT	Below 1.8%

Interpreting Liver Function Tests

Elevated AST and ALT (also called "transaminitis," "elevated liver enzymes," or "elevated LFTs") implies damage to liver cells of various causes—including alcoholic liver disease, hepatitis B or C, and nonalcoholic fatty liver disease.

Gastroenterologists tend to get less worked up about elevated enzymes than we do, and here are the usual definitions of mild/moderate/severe elevations:

- Mild elevation: Up to 5 times the upper limit of normal
- Moderate elevation: Between 5 and 10 times the upper limit of normal
- Marked elevation: More than 10 times the upper limit of normal

If liver enzymes are markedly elevated, this is a potential sign of acute liver failure (possibly due to ischemia or toxins) and your patient will need urgent evaluation by a specialist. For mild to moderate elevations, the next thing to do is to look at the patterns:

- Which is higher: AST or ALT?
  — If AST > ALT, with an AST/ALT ratio greater than 2, there's a 90% chance that the problem is alcoholic liver disease
  — If ALT > AST, with an ALT/AST ratio greater than 2, the problem may be drug-induced liver injury or nonalcoholic fatty liver disease
- GGT is fairly specific for alcoholic liver disease, and when it is elevated (along with an increased AST/ALT ratio) you can be even more confident that the issue is alcohol
- %CDT (carbohydrate-deficient transferrin) is an early marker of alcohol-induced hepatic injury that can be useful in identifying problems before they get worse; it can also detect under-reported drinking, and a positive result on this test suggests the patient has probably consumed 4 or more drinks a day for at least the past month
- Elevated alkaline phosphatase (ALP): Often due to bile duct obstruction or infiltrative liver disease impeding flow of bile out of the liver

To determine if your patient's liver is functioning poorly, check the following:

- Albumin and total protein: If low, it may be due to deficiencies in synthetic functioning, which would imply potential difficulties with synthesizing P450 enzymes
- Prothrombin time: If high, it may be due to poor synthesis of clotting factors

- Bilirubin: If high, it may be due to widespread damage to the biliary tree, which could be associated with decreased synthesis of various proteins and enzymes

Clinical Scenarios, Revisited

Scenario A: You advise the ED doc to go ahead and use chlordiazepoxide for the patient's detox, even though this drug has active metabolites. The patient has mild elevations of AST and ALT, consistent with mild hepatocellular damage due to alcohol use. But other labs, including albumin, bilirubin, and prothrombin time, are normal, and there is unlikely to be any impairment of liver functioning. Therefore, the patient should be able to adequately metabolize chlordiazepoxide and its active metabolites, and you anticipate that it will ensure a smoother detox.

Scenario B: You consult with the patient's gastroenterologist, who assures you that the patient does not have acute hepatitis and that her elevated enzymes have been chronic over the last two years. There are no signs of liver function impairment. Therefore, you feel comfortable that Vivitrol is not contraindicated in this patient, and, given the lethality of opioid use disorders, may even be life-saving.

CHAPTER 9

Excretion

DRUGS ARE EXCRETED FROM THE BODY in two ways: through the kidney (renal excretion) or through the bowel (fecal excretion). While most drugs used in medicine are primarily excreted through the kidney, many of the drugs we use in psychiatry are primarily excreted via the bowel. In this chapter, we'll discuss both mechanisms.

Renal Excretion

A Brief Kidney Lesson

The kidney is the body's great alchemist, turning blood into urine. It's composed of about one million nephrons, which are the working units of the organ, where the conversion of blood into urine takes place. In each nephron, the real action occurs in a special tuft of capillaries called the glomerulus. Think of it as a ball of string, in which the string is a long, twisted capillary. This ball sits inside a roundish cup called a Bowman's capsule, and as the heart pumps blood into the glomerulus, a filtrate is forced out of the capillaries and into the capsule. The pores in these capillaries are huge, so that basically everything filters out, including glucose, plasma, and most medications. What stays behind? Blood cells, big proteins, and any drugs that are bound to proteins.

Now, Bowman's capsule is like the basin of a water fountain with a pipe leading out of it. In the kidney, the pipe is not straight but is winding and convoluted. This leads us back to some of the more traumatic memories of Physiology 101, in which we were subjected to terms such as proximal convoluted tubule, distal convoluted tubule, collecting ducts, and—horror of horrors—the loop of Henle. Basically, they are all terms for different sections of one long twisty pipe carrying the filtrate from Bowman's capsule to the ureters, then to the bladder, and finally to the city plumbing.

Altogether, the bloodstream causes 180 liters of fluid per day to be filtered into Bowman's capsule and then into the tubules and ducts of the nephrons. That's more than 20 times the volume of blood. Luckily, the kidney has developed a fiendishly clever mechanism for reabsorbing 99% of the fluid, as well as glucose, vitamins, minerals, amino acids, and lots of ions, like sodium (Na+) and potassium (K+). How does it reabsorb all this stuff? Mostly, it's by forcing sodium ions out of the tubules and back into the bloodstream. Water and lots of other solutes passively follow, and, presto, we've gotten most of our blood back. So why have a kidney at all? What's the purpose of this elaborate process of filtering stuff out and then snatching most of it back in? Primarily it's to get rid of normal metabolic waste products, such as urea, but also to get rid of potentially toxic foreign products that we put into our system, like medications.

But how does the kidney prevent medications from getting reabsorbed along with everything else? That credit mostly goes to the tubules, which normally do not allow ionic compounds to pass through their membranes. Remember in Chapter 8 when we talked about biotransformation? The purpose of that, as you'll recall, is to turn lipophilic drugs into ionic, water-soluble versions of themselves. The ultimate plan is to have these ionic compounds get secreted into the kidney's tubules and trapped there, so that they exit with the urine.

Assessing Kidney Function

All the information above assumes that the kidney is healthy and working as it should. But sometimes kidney function gets impaired, and it's important for us to know how to order and interpret labs that can help us assess renal health. The usual renal function labs are blood urea nitrogen (BUN) and creatinine. To get a better understanding of how to interpret these labs, it's helpful to understand their origin.

BUN is a measure of how much urea is in your blood, and urea is ultimately a waste product of protein metabolism. Amino acids are metabolized to several products; one of them is ammonia (NH_3), which is toxic to the body and must be removed. The liver accomplishes this by orchestrating the urea cycle, in which ammonia combines with carbon dioxide to create urea (CH_4N_2O). Urea, while not as toxic as ammonia, becomes dangerous if the levels are too high (symptoms of excess urea include fatigue and delirium). So the kidney filters most of the urea out into its filtrate.

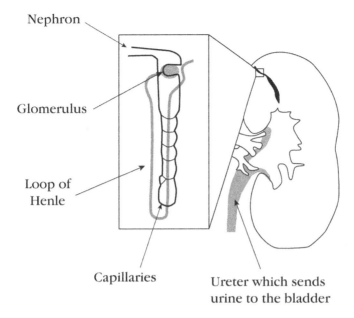

Nephron

Glomerulus

Loop of Henle

Capillaries

Ureter which sends urine to the bladder

FIGURE 9-1. Cross Section of Kidney

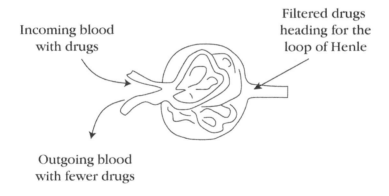

Incoming blood with drugs

Filtered drugs heading for the loop of Henle

Outgoing blood with fewer drugs

FIGURE 9-2. The Glomerulus

Urea is such an important and pungent part of the kidney filtrate that we've adapted its name to label the filtrate when it leaves our body: "urine."

Creatinine, meanwhile, comes from creatine phosphate, which is a source of the high-energy phosphates that we use in the form of ATP, which powers muscles. When creatine is phosphorylated, a byproduct is creatinine, which has no biological use and must be excreted by the kidney.

Getting back to renal labs, the normal range for BUN in many labs is 7–20 mg/dL, and the normal range for creatinine is 0.5–1.2 mg/dL. These values are also reported as a BUN/creatinine ratio, and the normal ratio is 10–20. Of the two values, the most accurate for measuring kidney function is creatinine. BUN is not as accurate because an elevated BUN can reflect dehydration, in which the kidney reabsorbs BUN as it tries to reabsorb more water from the urine. Dehydration does not cause creatinine to rise, because the kidney cannot reabsorb it.

Another lab we need to be familiar with is the glomerular filtration rate (GFR). Since the main function of the kidney is to filter stuff out of the blood, it stands to reason that the most important measure of kidney health is a measure of how well its filter is working. This is the GFR. The most accurate way to measure GFR is to do a creatinine clearance test, which requires a 24-hour urine collection to see how much creatinine your kidney can clear in 24 hours. But this is difficult to do, so usually we estimate the GFR based on the serum creatinine level. The lab results will report "eGFR" (estimated GFR). While creatinine level is a quick and dirty way to measure kidney function, the eGFR is more accurate.

The GFR is used to stage the severity of kidney disease, from stage 1 (mild) to stage 5 (renal failure). See the table below.

TABLE 9-1. Stages of Chronic Kidney Disease Based on Glomerular Filtration Rate (GFR)

Stage 1 (GFR 90 or more): Mild with normal renal function but other signs of kidney damage (eg, elevated albumin)
Stage 2 (GFR 60–89): Mild with impaired renal function
Stage 3 (GFR 30–59): Moderate
Stage 4 (GFR 15–29): Severe
Stage 5 (GFR less than 15): Renal failure, need for dialysis

How Does Kidney Impairment Affect Medication Doses?

A lot of people have kidney disease—in the US, about 8 million have chronic kidney disease, and 300,000 have end-stage renal disease (ESRD), meaning they are dependent on dialysis. So what do you do when you have a patient who has some degree of kidney disease? How does this affect your prescribing?

Generally speaking, most psychotropic medications are metabolized to inactive forms by the liver, and then excreted by the bowel into the feces. Because of this, as long as your kidney-impaired patient has an intact liver and GI system, you can prescribe most psychotropics as you would normally. However, for patients with severe or end-stage kidney disease (and who are on dialysis), there are a few special factors that you need to keep in mind, and here they are:

1. *Decreased protein binding.* Patients with kidney disease tend to have less albumin, due to reduced synthesis and leakage of protein in the urine. Many drugs we prescribe are highly protein bound, but it is only the unbound portion (the free fraction) that can have an effect on the body. Patients with less protein will tend to have a higher free fraction and therefore may need lower doses of some drugs.

2. *Decreased drug absorption.* Recall that a big part of drug absorption is the stomach giving pills an acid bath to dissolve them. ESRD patients often suffer "gastric alkalinization," which can interfere with efficient drug absorption.

3. *Increased volume of distribution.* ESRD patients often get edema because they aren't able to excrete their urine well. This causes a higher volume of distribution, which can dilute the concentration of drugs—and if so, you may have to increase doses.

In the end, you won't be able to guess whether dose adjustments are needed; you'll have to look this up in the drug's package insert. However, package inserts are often excessively cautious and will generally tell you to "reduce the dose in kidney disease," without specifying the severity of the kidney disease. This leads to clinicians reducing doses of meds even in patients with mild to moderate chronic kidney disease, which usually is not necessary. In fact, dosage adjustments are usually needed only in patients who have either stage 4 (severe) or stage 5 (dialysis-dependent) disease.

To make life easier for you, we've read a couple of comprehensive reviews of psychotropic drug dosing in kidney disease and have created the following handy tables for your quick reference. These tables clarify when dosing adjustments are needed—or not needed—in different degrees of kidney failure.

TABLE 9-2. No Dosage Adjustments Needed in Renal Impairment for the Following

Antidepressants
Fluoxetine
Fluvoxamine
Sertraline
Trazodone
Tricyclics (including amitriptyline, desipramine, and nortriptyline)
Antipsychotics
Aripiprazole
Asenapine
Haloperidol
Olanzapine
Quetiapine
Mood Stabilizers
Carbamazepine
Lamotrigine
Valproate
Anxiolytics/Hypnotics
Benzodiazepines
Zaleplon
Zolpidem

TABLE 9-3. Psychotropic Drugs: Recommended Dosing Adjustments in Kidney Disease

Medication	Mild to Moderate Renal Impairment (GFR > 30)	Severe Renal Impairment (GFR < 30)
Antidepressants		
Bupropion	None	Decrease dose by 50%
Duloxetine	None	Avoid
Escitalopram and citalopram	None	Decrease starting dose by 50% and titrate upward; be especially cautious with citalopram because of the risk of QTc prolongation
MAOIs	None	Avoid
Mirtazapine	None	Decrease dose
Paroxetine	None	Decrease dose by 50%
Venlafaxine	Decrease dose by 25%	Decrease dose by 50%

(table continues)

TABLE 9-3. Psychotropic Drugs: Recommended
Dosing Adjustments in Kidney Disease *(continued)*

Medication	Mild to Moderate Renal Impairment (GFR > 30)	Severe Renal Impairment (GFR < 30)
Antipsychotics		
Clozapine	None	Decrease dose
Lurasidone	Decrease dose	Decrease dose
Paliperidone	None	Decrease dose by 50%
Risperidone	None	Decrease dose by 50%
Ziprasidone	None	Avoid due to potential QTc interval changes
Mood Stabilizers		
Gabapentin	None	Decrease dose by 50%
Lithium	None	In ESRD patients, lithium is completely cleared by dialysis, so standard practice is to give a 600 mg dose after dialysis; a steady state will be maintained before the next dialysis session
Oxcarbazepine	None	Decrease dose

References

Cohen LM, Tessier EG, Germain MJ, Levy NB. Update on psychotropic medication use in renal disease. *Psychosomatics* 2004;45(1):34–48.

Baghdady NT, Banik S, Swartz SA, McIntyre RS. Psychotropic drugs and renal failure: translating the evidence for clinical practice. *Adv Therapy* 2009;26(4):404–424.

Ward S, Roberts JP, Resch WJ, Thomas C. When to adjust the dosing of psychotropics in patients with renal impairment. *Curr Psychiatr* 2016;15(8):60–66.

Lithium and the Kidney

Lithium travels through the bloodstream as a positive ion, Li+, which is a small molecule similar to sodium (Na+). When lithium reaches the kidney, it gets filtered into Bowman's capsule, and then into the nephron's system of tubules. Ordinarily the Li+ would stay in the tubules and eventually end up in the urine. But if Na+ transporters cannot find enough sodium to reabsorb, they'll sometimes settle for lithium. When taken to extremes, that reabsorption can lead to lithium toxicity, as in the situations below.

Dehydration. We're supposed to tell our patients on lithium to guard against dehydration. Why? Because when the kidney senses dehydration, it does what it can to reabsorb water. To accomplish this, it actively reabsorbs lots of Na+, and since Li+ and Na+ look similar to the kidney, it ends up sucking a lot of lithium back into the bloodstream, increasing lithium levels.

Diuretics

Hydrochlorothiazide is often used to treat hypertension. It does so by increasing sodium excretion in the kidney tubules, which leads to increased urination, decreased total body water, and therefore decreased blood pressure. The kidney doesn't particularly like to see such havoc being played with its fine-tuned homeostatic mechanism, and actively tries to compensate for the loss of sodium by retaining it elsewhere in the tubule system. But in snatching back up as much sodium as it can, the kidney indiscriminately snatches up a lot of lithium, causing an increase of up to 40% in lithium levels.

Angiotensin-converting enzyme (ACE) inhibitors, such as lisinopril and enalapril, also treat hypertension but through a different mechanism. They work by inhibiting the formation of angiotensin II (AG-II), which is normally a vasoconstrictor. If there is less AG-II around, arteries do not constrict as much, and blood pressure is reduced. How is this related to lithium? AG-II also promotes the release of a hormone called aldosterone, whose function is to cause the kidney to retain sodium. Since ACE inhibitors lower AG-II, they indirectly lower aldosterone, which in turn decreases the kidney's ability to retain sodium. The kidney compensates for this by trying to reabsorb sodium in other parts of the nephron, but it confuses lithium for sodium, causing higher levels of lithium.

Angiotensin receptor blockers (ARBs) such as losartan and valsartan can also increase lithium levels by preventing AG-II from binding to blood vessel receptors and lowering aldosterone.

NSAIDs raise lithium levels. It's not clear how, but the best guess is that they interfere with lithium's excretion by inhibiting prostaglandins. This problem is seen with ibuprofen, indomethacin, naproxen, and the COX-2 selective NSAID Celebrex—in fact, it's seen with all NSAIDs except aspirin and possibly sulindac. On average, the NSAIDs raise lithium levels by 20%, but the range is quite wide. To avoid surprises, cut the lithium dose by about 20% and recheck the level 5–10 days after starting an NSAID (or lower the dose more if the patient is sensitive to high levels). Lithium levels tend to increase over 5–10 days after adding an NSAID, with levels returning to baseline within about 7 days after stopping one (Demler TL, *US Pharm* 2012;37(11):HS16–HS19).

Caffeine does the opposite of the processes we've reviewed so far—it can decrease lithium levels. How? Caffeine increases the GFR, causing us to urinate more and leading to indiscriminate losses of solutes, including lithium. There are cases of patients becoming manic after increasing caffeine intake, not because of the caffeine itself but because the caffeine significantly decreased their lithium levels. For a review of two such cases, see the *Drug Interactions Casebook* by Neil Sandson (American Psychiatric Publishing; 2003).

Does Lithium Damage the Kidney?

About 10%–20% of patients on long-term lithium treatment experience some degree of renal insufficiency.

One study examined 114 psychiatric outpatients who had been taking lithium continuously for at least four years. Twenty-four (21%) of these patients exhibited the "creeping creatinine" phenomenon, with levels gradually reaching the 1.5 level, which is the standard cutoff point for the diagnosis of renal impairment. Most of these patients did not show this sign of renal impairment until 10–15 years of lithium treatment (Lepkifker E et al, *J Clin Psychiatry* 2004;65(6):850–856). A more recent review found that for people taking lithium on a chronic basis, renal function declines at a rate about 30% faster than what would be expected with typical aging.

The positive spin on these findings is that the majority of patients (around 80%) on long-term lithium treatment showed no signs of renal impairment whatsoever. Furthermore, in half of the patients with renal problems, the creatinine elevations reversed with simple dosage reductions.

Another way to reduce the renal risk is by dosing lithium once at night. This strategy worked in two long-term studies and one randomized trial, and it also reduces the risk of polyuria, which is one of the most common side effects on lithium (Schoot TS et al, *Eur Neuropsychopharmacol* 2020;31:16–32). Most cases of polyuria are benign, but a severe case may mean that lithium is causing nephrogenic diabetes insipidus (NDI). This syndrome happens when lithium alters the renal tubules in ways that make it hard for the kidneys to concentrate urine. The frequent urination is hard to live with, but the changes in the tubules also raise the risk of future renal impairment. NDI is diagnosed by testing urine osmolality, urine sodium, serum sodium, serum creatinine, and a 24-hour urine for volume.

Oddly, the way to treat patients who have severe polyuria and who need to remain on lithium is to give them a potassium-sparing diuretic, a medication that is usually used to *increase* urine production. How does this paradoxical remedy work? Basically, the diuretic starts in the usual way, by limiting sodium reabsorption, thereby increasing urine volume. The body then notices that it has less fluid in it, and this reduces the pressure at the glomerulus, causing a lower GFR. The kidney then responds to this by saying "Uh oh, we're running low on fluid, so let's decrease urine output"— leading, finally, to the desired outcome of less polyuria.

The best diuretic to use is the potassium-sparing diuretic amiloride, which is started at 5 mg/day. Amiloride works within 3 weeks and is one of the few diuretics that do not raise lithium levels. Amiloride is best managed through consultation with the medical team because it carries a risk of hyperkalemia, particularly in patients with renal insufficiency or diabetes.

Renal Monitoring on Lithium

While individual practice varies, most psychiatrists will check BUN/creatinine at least yearly, sometimes more frequently than that. What should you do if you see creatinine creeping up? If it's mild (less than 1.5 mg/dL), you can follow it and continue the lithium (while lowering the dose as much as possible). If creatinine gets to 1.5 or higher, you should refer to a nephrologist for consultation—who will likely ask that you discontinue the lithium. When you discontinue lithium, do two things. First, start your replacement mood stabilizer before tapering off the lithium. Second, taper the lithium very slowly—over at least 3 months—in order to decrease the risk of a relapse.

Biliary Excretion

While the kidney gets most of the glory when it comes to excreting drugs, in psychiatry biliary excretion is just as important as renal excretion—if not more so. Here's how it works:

1. Drugs go to the liver where they are metabolized in Phase I and/or Phase II reactions.
2. From the liver, the metabolites either go into the bloodstream to the kidney, or go directly into the hepatobiliary system.

3. The hepatobiliary system begins with small branching bile ducts within the liver that converge into the right and left hepatic ducts, and then into the common hepatic duct.
4. The common hepatic duct is joined with the cystic duct from the gallbladder (where bile is stored between meals) to form the common bile duct.
5. The common bile duct empties into the duodenum, which is the first part of the small intestine.
6. Finally, all the drug metabolites join with other waste to form feces, which eventually is excreted.

See the diagram below.

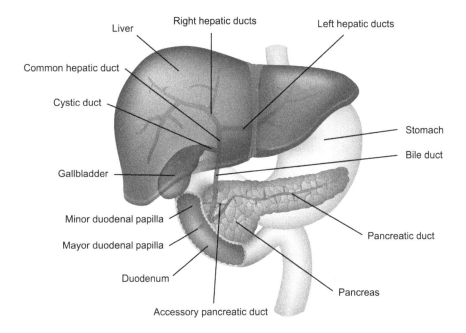

FIGURE 9-3. Biliary Anatomy

What happens when biliary excretion is impaired? Drugs like hydroxyzine that rely on biliary excretion will have poor elimination and should be avoided, and medications such as clonidine that act through enterohepatic circulation will have less predictable distribution.

Usually, problems with biliary excretion go hand in hand with liver disease. Refer back to Chapter 8 for a handy chart on drug dosing in these situations.

SECTION II

Drug Interactions

CHAPTER 10

Drug Interactions

*"!!! Warning: Use with caution. Modafinil may decrease the level
of olanzapine by affecting hepatic enzyme CYP1A2 metabolism"*
—Anonymous, drug interaction software

IF YOUR EHR CONSTANTLY INTERRUPTS you with messages like
the one above, you may be suffering from alert fatigue. We're here to help.
Only a few drug interactions really matter in psychiatry. The rest are rare,
theoretical, or simply iron themselves out on their own as we adjust the
dose based on the patient's response.

Theoretical interactions are the ones that show up in a petri dish but
don't necessarily pan out in the human body. It may be that the interaction
is too weak to change a drug's levels, or that it only affects one of several
pathways that a drug is metabolized through. In this book, we'll focus on
interactions that have demonstrated their relevance in human studies. We'll
also tell you how to adjust a dose to correct for an interaction, but keep in
mind those adjustments are just rough approximations. The bottom line is
not the numbers but your patient's response.

The Language of Drug Interactions

There are two types of drug interactions: *pharmacokinetic* and *pharmacodynamic*. Pharmacokinetic interactions are the ones that change drug levels,
whether through absorption, hepatic metabolism, entry into the CNS, or
excretion. We'll start with those and then move on to pharmacodynamic
interactions, which involve all the things that drugs do to the brain and
body, from therapeutic to adverse effects.

To understand pharmacokinetics, a little terminology is in order:

Substrate. A *substrate* is a drug that is metabolized by a particular
enzyme system. Thus, for example, tricyclics and beta blockers are both
substrates of the CYP2D6 enzyme system, because they are both metabolized by that system.

Inhibition. *Inhibition* happens when two drugs compete for the same metabolic enzyme. One drug (the inhibitor) binds more tightly to the enzyme than the other drug, and the *victim* drug then gets stuck in a game of metabolic musical chairs as it scurries around looking for an enzyme system to break it down. This leads, rather quickly, to higher drug levels than otherwise. To complicate things a bit, some drugs specialize in "non-competitive" inhibition, which is a shameless act of sabotage in which the aggressor drug is not a substrate of an enzyme but binds to it anyway, purely in order to disable it. The results are the same as in competitive inhibition—higher levels of the substrate.

Induction. *Induction* happens when the "inducing" drug stimulates the production of extra enzymes. If your patient is taking a medication that is metabolized by those same enzymes, then this medication will be broken down more rapidly than normal, leading to lower-than-predicted levels. Unlike inhibition, induction doesn't kick in right after the patient takes the inducing drug. Instead, it takes 1–3 weeks. Why? Because it takes this long for the liver to produce these extra enzymes. Think of it like a garden. You can tear down the plants pretty quickly (inhibition), but it takes a long time to grow new ones (induction).

Reversal. The levels of a victim drug (the substrate) also change after a patient stops an inducer or an inhibitor. This is called *reversal* of induction or inhibition. An example is a patient on alprazolam who stops fluvoxamine, which was raising alprazolam's level by inhibiting its breakdown. Once the patient stops the fluvoxamine, the CYP3A4 enzymes start breaking down more alprazolam, leading to a drop in alprazolam levels and a possible panic attack for the patient. The opposite happens when an inducer is stopped, as in the case of a patient on clozapine who finally quits smoking. We'll discuss how to manage this smoking interaction in Chapter 14.

Prodrugs. Some drugs are inert and don't do anything until they are converted to an active metabolite by the enzyme system. These are called *prodrugs*, and you may need to engage in a little reverse psychology to understand the interactions around them. In the prodrug world, inhibitors lower the therapeutic levels and inducers raise them. It's the opposite of what we normally expect, because an inhibitor blocks the conversion of the prodrug into its therapeutic metabolite.

Codeine, tramadol (Ultram), and hydrocodone (Vicodin) are prodrugs whose active forms can be blocked by antidepressants. These opioids have little analgesic effect until they are converted by CYP2D6 into morphine (from codeine), hydromorphone (from hydrocodone), or desmethyltramadol (from tramadol). Medications that block CYP2D6 can prevent that activation. The result is more pain and, if the interaction is missed, the risk that your patient will be mistaken for a drug seeker when they ask their physician to raise the dose.

Patients who are metabolizers at CYP2D6 are also prone to this analgesic-blocking effect, but there's a secret that can help you identify these patients without having to order an expensive genetic test. Have any of your patients ever listed "codeine" as a drug allergy? The prodrug in codeine causes lots of side effects (itching, nausea, headache, fatigue, and anticholinergic effects) but no analgesic effects. So if their experience with codeine was a lot of side effects—all pain, no gain—they may be a poor metabolizer at CYP2D6.

Another important prodrug is tamoxifen, which is converted by CYP2D6 into endoxifen, the active form of the drug that prevents recurrences of breast cancer. CYP2D6 inhibitors, particularly paroxetine, fluoxetine, and bupropion, can prevent that activation and thereby raise the risk of cancer.

In psychiatry the main prodrugs are lisdexamfetamine (Vyvanse), a difficult-to-abuse psychostimulant; gabapentin enacarbil (Horizant), a version of gabapentin that's approved in restless legs syndrome; and the long-acting injectable aripiprazole lauroxil (Aristada). None of these depend on hepatic metabolism to convert into their active forms, and we're not aware of any drug interactions that block their activation.

Active metabolites. Sometimes both the parent drug and its metabolite have active effects. The result is a kind of endogenous polypharmacy where the patient is effectively taking two or more drugs—the parent drug and the active metabolite—that may have overlapping or different effects. Drug makers often get fixated on active metabolites of drugs that are about to go off-patent.

For example, desvenlafaxine (Pristiq) is the active metabolite of venlafaxine (Effexor) and was introduced by Wyeth as Effexor was going generic. Whether desvenlafaxine has any advantages over venlafaxine is a matter of ongoing debate. Eszopiclone (Lunesta) has an active metabolite, S-desmethylzopiclone, that is more anxiolytic and less sedating than the parent drug. That might explain why eszopiclone worked in augmentation trials of generalized anxiety disorder and major depression, but other z-hypnotics did not (Pollack M et al, *Arch Gen Psychiatry* 2008;65(5):551–562).

Active metabolites complicate drug interactions because inducers and inhibitors may raise one drug while lowering the other. That means you can't simply correct for the interaction by raising or lowering the dose. With some drugs, like clozapine, you can check the levels of the parent drug and its active metabolite. Outside of that, the only solution is to watch closely and avoid this quagmire as much as possible. We'll learn how to do that when adding bupropion to SSRIs in the next chapter.

Keeping Up With Drug Interactions

No textbook of drug interactions is complete. This book will teach you the principles, but to apply them in practice you'll need an electronic database that keeps up with the growing pharmacopeia. The two that stand out are Lexi-Interact and Epocrates, which took first and second place for accuracy in a study that compared their results to those of a research pharmacist. The pharmacist was armed with four databases, including access to digital libraries of medical journals (Kheshti R et al, *J Res Pharm Pract* 2016;5(4):257–263).

1. **Lexi-Interact** is available online, through the Lexicomp app, or as part of an UpToDate subscription. Several studies have rated Lexi-Interact higher than its close competitor, Micromedex.
2. **Epocrates** came in second place, but is free with registration. It's also a good resource for finding out which tablet sizes and formulations are currently available.

Putting It All Together

Your patient comes in on multiple medications, and you are ready to check for interactions. Start by running the patient's medications through one of the aforementioned electronic databases. They tend to over-report interactions, so if nothing shows up, you are probably clear. If you get the message that one drug may lower the levels of another, you probably have a pharmacokinetic interaction on your hands and you may need to adjust the dose—that is, unless that interaction is purely theoretical, existing in a test tube but rarely seen in the human body. Other messages might warn of a pharmaco*dynamic* interaction, such as serotonin syndrome with an SSRI and a migraine medicine, or "neurotoxicity" with lithium and an antipsychotic. In Chapter 15 we'll highlight the pharmacodynamic interactions you really need to be wary of (as a hint, you can usually ignore the two examples just mentioned).

Getting back to the pharmacokinetic interactions, what if the interaction you've been warned of is a meaningful one and the medication you are about to add is likely to induce or inhibit the metabolism of another drug? You'll need to adjust that victim drug, but not just yet. Remember, inhibitors take a few days to kick in, while inducers take 2–4 weeks before they cause the victim's levels to fall.

For example, if you're adding valproate (an inhibitor) to lamotrigine, gradually cut the lamotrigine dose in half over the next 3 days. When adding carbamazepine (an inducer) to lamotrigine, gradually double the lamotrigine dose over the next 2 weeks. Exactly how fast you should act depends on the risks of shooting too high (side effects) or too low (loss of efficacy).

What about when you stop the offending drug? Generally, it takes the same amount of time for the effects to go away as it did for them to come on, which means they go away faster for inhibitors and slower for inducers. One exception is smoking. It only takes about 3 days for cigarette smoke to become a clinically meaningful inducer, and the reversal of that induction only takes about a week.

The adjustments we just gave for lamotrigine are pretty standard and available in the *PDR*, but for other medications the conversion is less precise. Throughout this book, we'll provide estimates from the available research. When the correction factor is unknown, use the table below.

TABLE 10-1. How to Adjust a Victim Drug

Type of Interaction	Dosage Adjustment
Strong inhibitor	Multiply target dose by 0.25–0.5
Moderate inhibitor	Multiply target dose by 0.7–0.8
Strong inducer	Multiply target dose by 2–4

Here's how to use the table. Suppose you want to start lurasidone (Latuda) in schizophrenia, an antipsychotic that is primarily metabolized through CYP3A4. Your patient is taking St. John's wort, a strong 3A4 inducer. Instead of aiming for, say, a daily dose of lurasidone 80 mg, you may need to aim higher, by 2–4 times that amount (160–320 mg). You should still start out with your usual titration, however, and adjust the dose by the patient's response, as these things are not 100% predictable. Suppose instead the patient has HIV and is taking ritonavir, which is a strong inhibitor of 3A4. Here you would lower the target lurasidone dose by 0.25–0.5 (from 80 mg to 20–40 mg). In this case, we would also recommend slowing down the titration. Why? The main goal of titration is to prevent premature dropout from side effects like akathisia. It's the inhibitors that raise those stakes, so we err on the side of caution, titrating slowly in their presence.

There's one caveat to those corrections. If a medication is a substrate of multiple enzymes, chances are that inhibitors will not increase its level very much, because the other enzymes will take over for the inhibited one. The moderating effect of multiple enzymes doesn't apply when the other drug is an inducer, however, because a single supercharged enzyme can chew up a substrate quickly even while other enzyme systems are sitting around and yawning. The moderating effect also doesn't apply when an inhibitor blocks multiple enzymes, as when the pan-inhibiting SSRIs (fluoxetine and fluvoxamine) cause tricyclic levels to rise.

A Short List of What You Really Need to Know

The critical interactions to pay attention to are the strong inducers and inhibitors in the table below. These can change the serum levels of other meds by 2- to 4-fold, both the medications that you prescribe and the ones on the medical side. In general, the higher the dose, the stronger the inhibition or induction.

TABLE 10-2. Inhibitors and Inducers to Watch For

Strong Inhibitors That Increase Other Drugs	Strong Inducers That Decrease Other Drugs
Valproate	Carbamazepine
Bupropion, duloxetine, nefazodone, fluvoxamine, paroxetine, fluoxetine, and high-dose sertraline (≥ 150 mg/day)	St. John's wort
Asenapine	Tobacco smoke
Grapefruit juice	

Your patients will appreciate it when you anticipate strong interactions ahead of time. In one study, 30% of patients developed significant extrapyramidal side effects after fluoxetine was added to their risperidone. The reason? Fluoxetine raises risperidone levels through CYP inhibition, and the resulting akathisia was intolerable (Spina E et al, *J Clin Psychopharma-col* 2002;22(4):419–423). Among the most critical interactions are those with victim drugs possessing a narrow therapeutic window, like warfarin or phenytoin. Even moderate interactions with those drugs can have toxic effects (see table below).

TABLE 10-3. Toxic Drug Interactions in Psychiatry

Medication	Potentially Raised By[1]	Toxic Effects
Benzos	**CYP3A4 inhibitors** (see below) raise alprazolam and triazolam. **Valproate** can raise diazepam and lorazepam. Fluoxetine, amiodarone, and cimetidine inhibit multiple enzymes and can raise some benzos.	Falls, cognitive problems, respiratory depression.
Carbamazepine	**CYP3A4 inhibitors.** **Azole antifungals, anti-retrovirals,** pimozide, diltiazem, verapamil, cimetidine, grapefruit juice, and cipro-/norfloxacin.	Coma, respiratory depression, seizures, arrhythmia, anticholinergic effects.
Lithium	**Thiazide diuretics** (HCTZ), **ACE inhibitors** (-prils), **angiotensin receptor blockers** (-sartans), NSAIDs, antibiotics (eg, tetracyclines, levofloxacin).	Renal failure, cerebellar damage, arrhythmias, coma, seizures. Past toxicity is not a contraindication for future lithium trials.
Trazodone	**CYP3A4 and 2D6 inhibitors.** **Azole antifungals, fluoxetine, paroxetine, pimozide,** diltiazem, verapamil, cimetidine, grapefruit juice, **anti-retrovirals,** and **antibiotics** (cipro- and norfloxacin).	Sedation with CYP3A4 inhibitors. CYP2D6 inhibitors may raise levels of mCPP, a metabolite that can cause depression, anxiety, and hallucinations.
Tricyclics	**CYP2D6 inhibitors.** **Fluoxetine, paroxetine,** sertraline at ≥ 150 mg, bupropion, **duloxetine, asenapine,** phenothiazines (chlorpromazine, perphenazine, thioridazine), **pimozide, quinidine, ritonavir.**	Cardiac arrest, arrhythmias, respiratory depression, seizures, hallucinations, hyperthermia.

[1]Strong inhibitors are in bold

Most other drug interactions are in the mild to moderate range. They won't cause serious problems, but understanding them can help fine-tune your dosing. For example, the usual target dose for quetiapine in bipolar depression is 300 mg/day, but lamotrigine lowers quetiapine a little, so you could push it to 400 mg/day when using the two together.

Protein Binding: Can We Finally Forget About It?

There's been a long-standing debate about the clinical relevance of "protein binding." Many drugs latch onto proteins in the bloodstream. This lowers the drug's effectiveness, because only the unbound fraction can actually have a biological effect. It can also cause surprising side effects, as when a newly prescribed drug with a higher affinity for a particular protein displaces the existing drug, causing a sudden rise in the biologically active, unbound fraction of the old drug.

While all this makes sense, it turns out that there are very few situations in which protein binding has a clinically significant effect on serum levels of medications, at least for the medications that psychiatrists are likely to prescribe. A review of this problem concluded that it only became significant with certain antibiotics prescribed on an intensive care unit (Roberts JA et al, *Clin Pharmacokinet* 2013;52(1):1–8). Most changes in unbound fractions caused by competing drugs are relatively minor, and any excess unbound drug tends to get metabolized and eliminated before it can cause toxicity. An exception is aspirin, which can raise free valproate levels by 10%–40%.

Outside of the psychotropics, there are a few protein-bound medications to look out for that have a narrow therapeutic window: warfarin, digoxin, and phenytoin. These can be displaced by psychiatric drugs that have high protein binding, namely duloxetine, fluoxetine, paroxetine, sertraline, nortriptyline, clozapine, haloperidol, valproate, and a few benzodiazepines (chlordiazepoxide, diazepam, and lorazepam). The best approach is to avoid prescribing these drugs together, but if you have to use them you'll need to watch for signs of toxicity as well as warn your patient and the other provider (Table 10-4).

TABLE 10-4. Protein-Bound Meds to Watch for

Protein-Bound Medication	Signs of Toxicity
Warfarin (Coumadin)	Bleeding, bruising, or signs of internal bleeding (dark stools from a GI bleed, acute headache from hemorrhagic stroke); elevated prothrombin time
Digoxin	Nausea and vomiting; low energy; cardiac arrhythmias or heart failure
Phenytoin	Ataxia; nystagmus; hypertrophy of the gums

Changes in free fractions of drugs can cause confusion when you order serum drug levels. Generally, the lab reports the sum of both the bound and the unbound medication. But what if the unbound portion is unusually high? That can happen when patients are taking a protein-bound drug that competes with the medication or when their albumin levels are low. To clarify the problem, order a "free fraction" serum level of the drug.

Now that you've got the basic concepts of pharmacokinetic interactions down, let's look at how they play out in the big three classes of psychiatric medications: antidepressants, antipsychotics, and mood stabilizers.

CHAPTER 11

Drug Interactions: Antidepressants

EVER WONDER HOW PSYCHIATRISTS GOT interested in the CYP system? It goes back to the early 1980s, when a few brave clinicians ventured into uncharted territory: the antidepressant combination. This kind of practice had been shunned for years because the only antidepressants available were MAOIs and tricyclics, and combining these has a dangerous tendency to cause serotonin syndrome.

The second-generation antidepressants provided a safer playing field to test out drug combinations, first with trazodone in 1981 and later with bupropion (Wellbutrin) and fluoxetine (Prozac). When tricyclic antidepressants were combined with these newcomers, patients got better without serotonin syndrome, but they soon ran into a new problem. Bupropion and the early SSRIs are strong inhibitors at enzymes that metabolize the tricyclics, particularly CYP2D6, and the consequences of this inhibition are potentially fatal. In this chapter, we'll look at the CYP drug interactions that you need to know when prescribing antidepressants, starting with the SSRIs.

SSRIs

Three SSRIs are strong CYP inhibitors that raise the levels of other medications:
- Fluoxetine (Prozac) is a strong inhibitor at CYP2D6 and 2C19
- Fluvoxamine (Luvox) is a strong inhibitor at CYP1A2, 2C19, 3A4, and 3A5
- Paroxetine (Paxil) is a strong inhibitor only at CYP2D6

Sertraline (Zoloft) is also a strong inhibitor at CYP2D6, but only at doses of 150 mg or greater. That leaves the "-prams," citalopram (Celexa) and escitalopram (Lexapro), as the only SSRIs that don't significantly disrupt the CYP system. However, while the -prams may not cause major CYP interactions, they are *victims* of CYP2C19 inhibitors. That victimization led the FDA to restrict citalopram's dose to 20 mg/day in patients who are taking a CYP2C19 inhibitor or are poor metabolizers at that enzyme, as well as in any patient over age 60. The reason is that citalopram has a high risk of prolonging the QTc interval, and this risk rises as the serum level or the patient's age goes up. Escitalopram is also vulnerable to this interaction, but it doesn't cause as much trouble for the QTc, so the FDA let it off the hook.

TABLE 11-1. Psychotropics That Inhibit CYP Enzymes

CYP Enzyme	Mild-Moderate Inhibitors	Strong Inhibitors
CYP2D6	Bupropion, fluvoxamine, tranylcypromine, venlafaxine, vilazodone, tricyclics (doxepin, desipramine, imipramine); clozapine, risperidone, phenothiazines (chlorpromazine, perphenazine, thioridazine); curcumin (turmeric)	Fluoxetine, paroxetine, sertraline at ≥ 150 mg, duloxetine; asenapine, pimozide; cannabidiol (CBD oil)
CYP1A2	Curcumin, caffeine	Fluvoxamine, viloxazine (Qelbree)
CYP3A4	Desvenlafaxine, milnacipran; clozapine, haloperidol, ziprasidone	Fluvoxamine, nefazodone; curcumin
CYP2C19	Sertraline; modafinil, armodafinil	Fluoxetine, fluvoxamine, clomipramine, imipramine

Fluvoxamine: The Great Inhibitor

Fluvoxamine raises many drug levels as a potent pan-inhibitor throughout the CYP system, but most of these interactions are not cause for alarm. Extensive post-marketing surveillance of fluvoxamine has not revealed a great deal of adverse events. For example, in one study, fluvoxamine nearly doubled alprazolam levels, yet there was no increase in sedation or memory problems. The higher alprazolam levels did slow down reaction times on cognitive tests of repetitive tasks, however (Fleishaker JC and Hulst LK, *Eur J Clin Pharmacol* 1994;46(1):35–39).

Potentially serious interactions with fluvoxamine include clozapine, clomipramine, theophylline, and warfarin. High levels of theophylline and warfarin can be fatal, while increases in clomipramine and clozapine can cause sedation, seizures, and arrhythmias.

The clozapine story is made more complex by an active metabolite. Fluvoxamine blocks the conversion of clozapine into norclozapine, a metabolite that is responsible for many of clozapine's adverse effects. When done carefully, this interaction can be harnessed to improve clozapine's tolerability. We'll get to that in the next chapter.

Other medications that might rise to dangerous levels when taken with fluvoxamine include ramelteon (Rozerem), a hypnotic that may be overly sedating at high levels, and flibanserin (Addyi), a medication for female sexual dysfunction that can make people faint when its levels go too high.

While fluvoxamine inhibits CYP1A2, other medications induce this enzyme, like carbamazepine and the modafinils. If those inducers are ever combined with a strong inhibitor like fluvoxamine, you can't assume that the effects will cancel each other out. Watch carefully, as it could go either way.

TABLE 11-2. Medications Raised by Fluvoxamine

Psychiatric	Nonpsychiatric
Antidepressants: Duloxetine, mirtazapine, amitriptyline, clomipramine, imipramine **Antipsychotics:** Asenapine, clozapine, haloperidol, olanzapine **Hypnotics:** Melatonin, ramelteon **Other:** Caffeine, propranolol, flibanserin	Acetaminophen, cyclobenzaprine, estradiol, mexiletine, naproxen, ondansetron, phenacetin, riluzole, ropivacaine, tacrine, theophylline, tizanidine, verapamil, warfarin, zileuton, zolmitriptan

Tricyclics

Tricyclics are often the victim of CYP drug interactions. Inducers can render them ineffective, but inhibitors are the bigger problem as high levels of tricyclics can have serious consequences: hyperthermia, respiratory depression, delirium, seizures, arrhythmias, and cardiac arrest.

SSRIs and bupropion are common causes of high tricylic levels, but the problem is widespread enough that it's worth checking for drug interactions when combining tricyclics with other medications. If an inhibitor is already on board, add the tricyclic in gradually. For example, start with half the dose, raise it slowly, and aim for half the usual target dose. Once you reach the target, fine-tune the dose based on the patient's response. With amitriptyline, imipramine, and nortriptyline, you can also check the patient's blood level to see if it is in the therapeutic range (Table 11-3).

TABLE 11-3. Therapeutic Levels of Antidepressants

Medication	Therapeutic Serum Level
Amitriptyline	150–300 ng/mL
Imipramine*	175–350 ng/mL (for the sum of imipramine and its metabolite desipramine)
Nortriptyline*	50–150 ng/mL
Duloxetine	Above 58 ng/mL
Trazodone	Above 650 ng/mL
Venlafaxine	125–400 ng/mL (for the sum of venlafaxine and its metabolite desmethylvenlafaxine)

*These therapeutic windows are well established

Trazodone

What could go wrong when a sedating antidepressant is used for sleep? Trazodone may not cause people to drive or cook in an amnestic state like the z-hypnotics and benzodiazepines can. But it *can* cause orthostatic falls and leave patients a little groggy and cognitively impaired the next day, not to mention the possibility of priapism (a painful enlarged erection of the penis or painfully engorged clitoris). Those risks are heightened by CYP3A4 inhibitors, including grapefruit and a host of medications that prolong trazodone's half-life by blocking its main route of elimination (Table 11-4).

TABLE 11-4. Common 3A4 Inhibitors

CYP3A4 Inhibitors	Medications They Can Raise
Antidepressants: Desvenlafaxine, milnacipran, fluvoxamine, nefazodone	Carbamazepine, trazodone, alprazolam, triazolam
Antipsychotics: Clozapine, haloperidol, pimozide, ziprasidone	
Other: Azole antifungals, antiretrovirals, cimetidine, ciprofloxacin, diltiazem, norfloxacin, verapamil, curcumin (turmeric), grapefruit juice	

VERDICT

If your patient calls with unusual fatigue the day after taking trazodone, first lower the dose. If that doesn't work, check for drug and grapefruit interactions, and consider the possibility that the patient may be a poor metabolizer at CYP3A4.

TABLE 11-5. Common 2D6 Inhibitors

CYP2D6 Inhibitors	Medications They Can Raise
Strong inhibitors: Duloxetine, fluoxetine, paroxetine, sertraline at ≥ 150 mg; asenapine, pimozide, quinidine, ritonavir, cannabidiol (CBD oil) **Mild-moderate inhibitors:** Bupropion, fluvoxamine, tranylcypromine, venlafaxine, vilazodone, tricyclics (doxepin, desipramine, imipramine); clozapine, risperidone, phenothiazines (chlorpromazine, perphenazine, thioridazine); curcumin (turmeric)	**Antidepressants:** Mirtazapine, tricyclics, some SSRIs and SNRIs (duloxetine, escitalopram, fluoxetine, fluvoxamine, levomilnacipran, paroxetine) **Antipsychotics:** Aripiprazole, brexpiprazole, iloperidone, risperidone **Other:** Atomoxetine, deutetrabenazine

Metabolic Polypharmacy

Polypharmacy is generally frowned upon, especially when two drugs from the same class are combined. But the metabolic system creates these combinations even without a prescription by converting drugs into active metabolites. We've listed a few examples in Table 11-6 on the following page.

Drug interactions have unpredictable results when active metabolites are involved. Inducers will lower the level of the parent drug, but they may not render it ineffective because they simultaneously raise the active metabolite. Inhibitors, on the other hand, will cut off the active metabolite's production.

Here's how that might play out in practice. Your patient has recovered from depression on venlafaxine (Effexor) but has some residual anxiety. They start taking CBD oil on their own for the anxiety, but soon their depression worsens. You check on PubMed, but find no reports of worse depression with CBD—in fact, you even come across a few studies showing it can have anxiolytic effects. What is going on?

CBD oil is cannabidiol, a strong CYP2D6 inhibitor, so we'd expect it to raise venlafaxine. But it's also blocking the conversion of venlafaxine into another antidepressant, desvenlafaxine (Pristiq). It's likely that this metabolite, rather than venlafaxine, was responsible for the patient's recovery, and a reasonable next step is to switch to desvenlafaxine or stop the CBD.

Active metabolites can also muck up the picture in one of the oldest antidepressant augmentation strategies around: adding bupropion to an SSRI.

TABLE 11-6. Antidepressants With Active Metabolites

Parent Drug	Active Metabolites	Enzyme That Produces the Metabolite
Amitriptyline	Nortriptyline	2C19
Bupropion	Hydroxybupropion	2B6
Citalopram	Didesmethylcitalopram, desmethylcitalopram	2C19, 3A4
Clomipramine	Norclomipramine	2D6, 1A2
Doxepin	Nordoxepin	2C19
Escitalopram	Didesmethylcitalopram, desmethylcitalopram	2C19, 3A4
Fluoxetine	Norfluoxetine	2D6, 2C9
Imipramine	Desipramine	2C19
Mirtazapine	Desmethylmirtazapine, normirtazapine	1A2, 2D6, 3A4
Sertraline	Norsertraline, dasotraline	Multiple CYP enzymes
Venlafaxine	Desvenlafaxine	2D6

The Two Bupropions

In theory, adding bupropion to an SSRI creates the holy grail of antidepressants: a triple-reuptake inhibitor that works on serotonin, dopamine, and norepinephrine. Sounds good, but in well-designed clinical trials this strategy often falls flat. A drug interaction may explain why.

Bupropion is really two drugs. There's bupropion, and then there's its active metabolite hydroxybupropion, which is produced by the CYP2B6 enzyme (that's 2B6, not 2D6). Most SSRIs block this enzyme, resulting in higher levels of bupropion and lower levels of hydroxybupropion. In theory, this interaction could weaken bupropion's efficacy because hydroxybupropion's noradrenergic effects are about twice as potent as bupropion's.

Only two SSRIs are free of this CYP2B6 interaction: citalopram and escitalopram. That raises an intriguing possibility: Could bupropion augmentation work better with the "-pram" SSRIs? Maybe. No one has tested the idea directly, but it gets some support from the four large controlled trials of bupropion augmentation. When added to a -pram, bupropion augmentation was successful (the STAR*D trial) or at least worked on secondary outcomes (the CO-MED trial). When added to 2B6 inhibitors, it failed in both studies (the VAST-D trial and NCT00296517, a large industry-sponsored trial that never got published).

VERDICT

If you're going to combine bupropion with an SSRI, choose citalopram or escitalopram to avoid drug interactions that might diminish its antidepressant effects.

CHAPTER 12

Drug Interactions: Antipsychotics and Mood Stabilizers

Antipsychotics

WHEN IT COMES TO DRUG interactions, antipsychotics are often the victim but rarely the perpetrator. Antipsychotic blood levels are changed by many of the medications they are commonly paired with, such as SSRIs, carbamazepine, and valproate. Rather than memorize all these interactions, it's worth checking for them before you prescribe. It's also worth knowing the exceptions where you don't need to worry about CYP interactions. These friendlier neighbors that don't alter antipsychotic levels are lithium, lamotrigine, mirtazapine, vilazodone, vortioxetine, a few SNRIs (venlafaxine, desvenlafaxine, levomilnacipran), and the "-pram" SSRIs (citalopram and escitalopram).

The atypical antipsychotics don't tend to inhibit or induce the metabolic enzymes (with the exception of asenapine, which can double many medication levels through CYP2D6 inhibition). Nearly all atypical antipsychotics are lowered by carbamazepine, which can get in the way of augmentation strategies in bipolar disorder. Asenapine is the least affected by this interaction.

Should We Order Blood Levels of Antipsychotics?

Antipsychotic drug levels are sometimes used to check adherence, particularly when considering a trial of clozapine in schizophrenia. Clozapine is recommended after 2 failed antipsychotic trials, and the American Psychiatric Association recommends a blood level for at least one of those trials to confirm the patient was actually taking it.

Clozapine is also the antipsychotic whose serum levels are established enough to guide the dosing. In schizophrenia, the target range for clozapine is 250–350 ng/mL. Some patients require higher levels, but clozapine toxicity starts to kick in above 750 ng/mL. Clozapine's levels are usually reported along with its metabolite, norclozapine, which is responsible for many of clozapine's side effects. Ideally, the clozapine will be at least 1.5–2 times greater than norclozapine.

You may see therapeutic ranges listed for other antipsychotics, but few of these are backed by clinical studies, so they are more useful for checking adherence than optimizing the dose. Two exceptions are olanzapine (20–80 ng/mL) and haloperidol (1–10 ng/mL).

Clozapine, Quetiapine, and Their Nor- Metabolites

Many antipsychotics have active metabolites, but usually we don't know much about what those metabolites do. One exception is loxapine, which is metabolized to form the tetracyclic antidepressant amoxapine. Clozapine and quetiapine also form metabolites with interesting clinical properties.

Clozapine's metabolite norclozapine contributes to clozapine's side effects while adding little to the drug's therapeutic benefits. In theory, clozapine would be better tolerated if we blocked the enzyme that produces norclozapine, CYP3A4. That theory was successfully tested by adding 50 mg of fluvoxamine, a potent CYP3A4 inhibitor, to clozapine in a randomized, placebo-controlled trial of patients with schizophrenia. The clozapine dose was also lowered (from 300 to 100 mg/day) in the fluvoxamine group to account for the interaction. After 12 weeks, the fluvoxamine group had less weight gain, better insulin sensitivity, lower triglyceride levels, and fewer psychotic symptoms (Lu ML et al, *Schizophr Res* 2018;193:126–133).

Quetiapine is a structural derivative of clozapine and also produces an active metabolite through CYP3A4: norquetiapine (aka N-desalkylquetiapine). Norquetiapine doesn't have much in the way of antipsychotic effects, but it does have antidepressant properties, with serotonergic, noradrenergic, and dopaminergic effects that are more potent than the parent compound. Supporting this idea, higher norquetiapine levels are associated with better antidepressant effects on quetiapine, but also with a greater risk of manic switching. In practice, this means you'll need to be extra careful about CYP3A4 interactions with quetiapine. Inducers like carbamazepine, St. John's wort, and the modafinils could raise the antidepressant metabolite, while inhibitors could block its production.

Anticonvulsants

Three anticonvulsants are FDA approved in psychiatry, and all are used as mood stabilizers. Two of them, valproate and carbamazepine, are often the cause of drug interactions, while the third, lamotrigine, is often the victim of such interactions.

Carbamazepine

Carbamazepine (Equetro, Tegretol) is a strong inducer, meaning that it causes the liver to increase production of various metabolic enzymes, thereby decreasing levels of other drugs. It induces CYP1A2, 2C9, 2C19, 2A6, and 2B6, as well as the glucuronidation system that lamotrigine is metabolized through. But carbamazepine doesn't stop there. It also induces the enzyme that's responsible for its own metabolism, CYP3A4.

This means that your patient's carbamazepine level is going to fall by 30%–50% as CYP3A4 induction revs up. It takes a few weeks to induce an enzyme, while inhibition takes only a few days. To keep tabs on this trend, you should check carbamazepine levels at 3, 6, and 9 weeks after starting treatment, and expect the level to fall by 30%–50% during that time. Some of this decline is buffered, however, by the fact that carbamazepine has an active metabolite—carbamazepine-10,11-epoxide—whose levels rise as the parent drug falls.

If getting a manic patient to check their labs every 3 weeks sounds like a tall order, take heart. Carbamazepine's serum levels do not necessitate the scientific precision of, say, lithium's, so it's best to let the patient's response guide the dose. Most patients arrive at a dose of 600–1200 mg/day, which corresponds to a serum level of 4–12 mcg/mL.

Autoinduction may also necessitate more frequent dosing because it shrinks carbamazepine's half-life from about 24 hours to 12 hours. In practice, however, the dosing schedule is best guided by tolerability.

Twice-a-day dosing reduces the dizziness and double vision that are associated with peak levels, and giving the bulk of the medicine in the evening reduces its sedative effects.

It also takes a few weeks for induction to impact the other drugs that carbamazepine interacts with. Those interactions are so numerous that some clinicians dismiss carbamazepine just to avoid the headache of managing them. But that's unfortunate, because carbamazepine is often just the right choice for patients with bipolar disorder who don't respond to—or can't tolerate—lithium or valproic acid.

A common misconception is that you can solve all your carbamazepine woes by simply substituting it with oxcarbazepine—the "kinder, gentler" analog of carbamazepine. In fact, oxcarbazepine *does* induce the CYP3A4 system, and even though it does so only about half as strongly as its cousin, that's still a potent-enough effect to render oral contraceptives ineffective.

Rather than avoiding carbamazepine, the better strategy is to look up the potential interactions and adjust the dose of the co-administered meds as needed. To save you from opening up your Epocrates app, Table 12-1 lists the medications whose levels are significantly lowered by carbamazepine; you may need to increase the dose of these meds to account for this effect. For example, lamotrigine doses need to be doubled on carbamazepine.

Most of these adjustments are approximate. If maintaining the level of another drug is critical, you can fine-tune your dosing by checking the serum level of the victim drug before adding carbamazepine, and then checking again a few weeks after adding it. We don't recommend trying this out if your patient is on oral contraceptives, because the risks are too high—better to either switch mood stabilizers or use a different method of contraception.

Patients will appreciate your efforts to stay the course with carbamazepine, as many find its side effects more favorable than other mood stabilizers in areas like weight gain, sedation, and metabolic effects. Oxcarbazepine is even better; it is 20%–40% less likely to cause side effects than carbamazepine. However, oxcarbazepine's gain in tolerability is usually outweighed by its lack of efficacy. In bipolar disorder, oxcarbazepine has more negative than positive trials (Vasudev A et al, *Cochrane Database Syst Rev* 2011;(12):CD004857).

TABLE 12-1. Medications Whose Levels Are Lowered by Carbamazepine

Huge (> 70% decrease in levels)	Aripiprazole, cariprazine, lurasidone, quetiapine; sertraline, trazodone
Major (50%–70% decrease in levels)	Brexpiprazole, clozapine, iloperidone, olanzapine, risperidone; lamotrigine, topiramate; mirtazapine, trazodone, vilazodone; z-hypnotics (eszopiclone, zaleplon, zolpidem)
Moderate (30%–50% decrease in levels)	Paliperidone, ziprasidone
Mild (20%–30% decrease in levels)	Asenapine, citalopram, escitalopram, paroxetine
Other (levels are lowered by variable or unknown degrees)	Benzodiazepines (alprazolam, clonazepam), tricyclic antidepressants, first-generation antipsychotics (chlorpromazine, fluphenazine, haloperidol, thiothixene), buprenorphine, bupropion, buspirone, levothyroxine, modafinils, methadone, methylphenidate, nefazodone, oxcarbazepine, valproate

Valproate

While carbamazepine tends to lower medication levels, valproate (Depakote) usually raises them. One of the most important valproate interactions is with lamotrigine, whose levels are doubled by valproate. High levels of lamotrigine raise the risk of serious rashes when starting the drug, so lamotrigine's titration schedule and target dose are cut in half when valproate is on board.

Other valproate interactions are more complex. Valproate tends to raise clozapine levels, unless the patient is a smoker, in which case it's more likely to lower those levels. It can also raise or lower risperidone levels, for reasons that are unclear. Through UGT2B15 inhibition, valproate can raise levels of the three benzodiazepines: lorazepam, temazepam, and oxazepam (these are the only benzos that are free of CYP interactions). NSAIDs like ibuprofen, naproxen, and aspirin can increase levels of free valproate by displacing it from serum protein.

TABLE 12-2. Medications Whose Levels Are Altered by Valproate

Decreased levels (usually by 30%–50%)	Asenapine, clozapine, olanzapine, risperidone
Increased levels (usually by 2-fold)	Quetiapine, lamotrigine, tricyclic antidepressants

Lamotrigine

Lamotrigine (Lamictal) is metabolized outside the CYP system through glucuronidation, and there it falls victim to the carbamazepine and valproate interactions described above. You'll sometimes hear that lamotrigine interferes with oral contraceptives, but actually it's the other way around. Oral contraceptives containing ethinyl estradiol and other estrogenic compounds lower lamotrigine by 30%–50% by inducing glucuronidation. Lamotrigine can lower levels of quetiapine by 20%–30% through an unclear mechanism. The typical quetiapine dose in bipolar depression is 300 mg/day, but you could go to 400 mg/day if lamotrigine is on board.

TABLE 12-3. Drugs That Decrease Levels of Oral Contraceptive Pills and Hormone Replacement Therapy

Carbamazepine
Oxcarbazepine
Modafinil, armodafinil
Topiramate

Lithium

Lithium has the narrowest therapeutic window in psychiatry. A serum level of 0.6–1.2 is therapeutic, while anything above 1.2 is potentially toxic. Lithium toxicity causes acute symptoms of imbalance, severe tremor, vomiting, slurred speech, and confusion, but its long-term implications are the real concern. Renal function declines with each toxic level, and lithium toxicity can damage the cerebellum, causing permanent problems with walking (ataxia). We reviewed ways to avoid toxicity in Chapter 9, and here we'll share some tips on managing lithium's drug interactions.

The main culprits are antihypertensives and NSAIDs, but it's worth checking any new medication that's added to your patient's list. Among the drugs that interact with lithium, thiazides have the strongest effect, raising lithium by 25%–50%, and angiotensin II antagonists have the weakest effect. However, the degree will vary by patient, so it's best to take a conservative approach and lower the lithium dose by 50% when an offending medication is added, then recheck the level in 5 days. Lithium levels can be monitored every 6–12 months in stable patients, but you may need to check more often if drug interactions are present, or if the patient is elderly or has an elevated creatinine.

TABLE 12-4. Lithium Levels

	Children and Adults	Geriatrics (≥ 65)	Treats
Low	0.1–0.5	0.1–0.3	Unclear; low levels may augment other mood stabilizers and might prevent dementia, suicide, and the progression of bipolar disorder
Medium	0.6–0.8	0.3–0.6	Depression (as monotherapy in bipolar depression, or as antidepressant augmentation in unipolar); this is also a good maintenance level to prevent episodes of mania or depression
High	0.8–1.2	0.6–0.8	Active mania
Toxic	> 1.2	Varies	Only causes harm

TABLE 12-5. Factors That Alter Lithium Levels

Raises Lithium	Lowers Lithium
Drug interactions: antihypertensives, diuretics, NSAIDs, and more (see Table 12-6)	**Drug interactions:** acetazolamide, xanthines (aminophylline, theophylline), mannitol
Dehydration	Caffeine
Aging	Active mania*
Renal slowing	Pregnancy
Low-sodium diet	Going off a low-sodium diet

*Lithium levels fall during active mania, possibly due to increased urination in the manic state

TABLE 12-6. Medications That Raise Lithium

Class	Examples
Thiazides and loop diuretics	The "-ides": bumetanide, chlorothiazide, furosemide, hydrochlorothiazide (potassium-sparing diuretics like amiloride and spironolactone are OK)
ACE inhibitors	The "-prils": benazepril, captopril, enalapril, lisinopril
Angiotensin II antagonists	The "-sartans": azilsartan, losartan, valsartan
NSAIDs and COX-2 inhibitors	**Over-the-counter:** ibuprofen, naproxen (aspirin is OK) **Prescription:** celecoxib, diclofenac, indomethacin, meloxicam (sulindac is usually OK)
Antibiotics	Metronidazole, tetracycline

NSAIDs create a unique dilemma because they are often taken as needed. In this case, have the patient lower their lithium dose by 30%–50% on the days they take the NSAID, and check the level on and off the NSAID to make sure it stays within a safe range. The NSAID sulindac (Clinoril) is preferred because it is the least likely to interact with lithium, but double-checking is still in order as there have been a few cases of lithium toxicity with sulindac.

In addition to the pharmacokinetic interactions listed in tables 12-5 and 12-6, there are two pharmacodynamic interactions that may raise flags when your patient brings their lithium script to the pharmacy. Lithium is reported to cause neurotoxicity (ie, stiffness, tremor, and mental status changes) when combined with antipsychotics. This concern has fizzled since it was first reported in the 1970s. With hindsight, it looks like the problems were due to the additive effects of the two drugs rather than a specific interaction between them (Kessel JB et al, *J Psychiatry Neurosci* 1992;17(1):28–30). The other concern is serotonin syndrome when lithium is combined with serotonergic antidepressants. This risk is real (lithium does have serotonergic properties) but extremely rare, and it only warrants caution when combining lithium with MAOIs.

Lithium and Salt

Though we've never heard of a patient getting manic from a pretzel binge, a sudden increase in dietary salt does cause lithium levels to fall. Likewise, shifting to a low-salt diet will cause a lithium spike and potentially dangerous toxicity. Low-salt diets are often recommended for high blood pressure, which poses an even greater risk of toxicity if a lithium-raising antihypertensive is added. Low-salt diets are also recommended to manage two side effects that can occur on lithium: edema and renal disease.

Another common problem with lithium is dehydration. Lithium levels rise as water leaves the body and the serum becomes more concentrated. Patients should know the risk factors for dehydration—alcohol, diarrhea, fever, systemic illness, and hot, sweaty days—and drink plenty of water during those times.

Hydration is also the first-line intervention for lithium toxicity. When a patient calls with severe imbalance, confusion, blurry vision, or myoclonic muscle jerks on lithium, send them to the emergency room to get their level checked. On the way there, have them drink a lot of water or—even better—an isotonic drink like Gatorade to flush the lithium out (patients can make their own isotonic solution by mixing ½ teaspoon of salt into 1 cup of warm water).

CHAPTER 13

Food and Drink Effects on Medications

FOOD INTERACTS WITH MEDICATION IN several ways:
- **Absorption.** Foods that alter gastric acidity or the rate of transport through the GI tract can change how medications are absorbed.
- **Bioactive compounds.** Some foods contain bioactive compounds that cause pharmacokinetic interactions (eg, grapefruit) or pharmacodynamic interactions (eg, tyramine-rich foods with MAOIs).

Food and Drug Absorption

Patients often want to know whether to take medications with meals or not. There are two parts to the answer. The first relates to comfort, while the second relates to the rate of absorption.

In terms of comfort, many patients experience nausea when they take psychiatric medications. For SSRIs, some of this comes from stimulation of serotonin receptors in the gut wall, a problem that won't go away by eating a snack with your medication. But there is also some local irritation, both with SSRIs and with other drugs, and taking medication during or right after a meal often helps.

What about drug absorption? How do meals affect this? Recall from Chapter 3 that drug absorption does not occur until medications pass through the stomach and into the small intestine. It therefore stands to reason that anything slowing the movement of content out of the stomach (known as "gastric emptying") would also slow down medication absorption. Food slows gastric emptying, because when the stomach distends with a meal it senses that it has to hold on to that meal for an extra 20 minutes or so to break it down with stomach acids. If there happen to be medications mixed in, those medications will have to wait for the stomach

125

TABLE 13-1. Psychiatric Medications Best Taken With Meals

	Medication	Instructions	Reason
Essential	Lurasidone (Latuda)	Take with ≥ 350-cal meal	Absorption drops 30%–70% if taken on an empty stomach
	Paliperidone (Invega)	Take with food	Food increases serum levels by 50%–60%
	Ziprasidone (Geodon)	Take with ≥ 500-cal meal	Absorption drops 50% if taken on an empty stomach
	Vilazodone (Viibryd)	Take with full meal	Absorption drops 50% if taken on an empty stomach
	Gabapentin enacarbil XR (Horizant)	Take with food at 5 pm	Absorption drops 25%–50% if taken on an empty stomach
	Gabapentin XR (Gralise)	Take with food in evening	Absorption drops 50% if taken on an empty stomach
Optional	Lithium	Take after a meal or with milk	Food mildly increases absorption and reduces nausea and diarrhea
	Sertraline (Zoloft)	Take consistently either with or without food	Food increases absorption
	Buspirone (Buspar)	Take consistently either with or without food	Food increases absorption 2-fold
	Propranolol	Take consistently either with or without food	High-protein meal increases absorption by 50%
	Atomoxetine (Strattera)	Take with food if nauseous	Food does not reduce absorption, but delays peak level by 3 hours
	Deutetrabenazine (Austedo)	Take with food	Food increases peak levels by 50%

to decide it is time to empty into the rest of the bowel. The bottom line is that if your patients want a drug to be absorbed as quickly as possible (for example, if they are eagerly waiting for the effects of a benzodiazepine), you should counsel them to take it on an empty stomach and drink plenty of water, which tends to speed transit time. For example, diazepam is delayed by 1 hour and its serum levels are lower when taken with a meal.

Interestingly, though, some drugs are absorbed faster *with* food, for reasons that are not entirely clear. Sertraline (Zoloft), for example, is absorbed faster after a meal, and the maximum concentration is increased

TABLE 13-2. Psychiatric Medications Best Taken on an Empty Stomach

	Medication	Instructions	Reason
Essential	Quetiapine XR (Seroquel XR)	Do not take within 1 hour of a heavy meal (≥ 300 cal)	Alcohol and high-fat meals cause the XR capsule to rapidly dump its dose, raising the risk of sedation and hypotension
	Asenapine (Saphris)	Allow pill to dissolve fully in mouth (10 minutes) before eating or drinking; do not swallow pill	Absorption drops 30% with food or drink; absorbed in the mouth, not in the gut
	Z-hypnotics (zolpidem, zaleplon, eszopiclone) Suvorexant (Belsomra), lemborexant (Dayvigo)	Do not take within 30 min of eating	Food delays the release by 1–2 hours
	Thyroid meds and tetracyclines	Take 1 hour away from food and other medications	Foods or meds with calcium or magnesium in them impair absorption
Optional	Nefazodone	Best to take away from food	Food lowers absorption by 20%
	All amphetamines (Adderall, Adzenys, Dexedrine, Evekeo, Mydayis, Vyvanse)	Avoid with acidic foods (fruit juice, sodas)	Decreased absorption
	Adderall XR	Best to take away from a large meal	Serum concentrations are lowered by up to 50% if taken with a large fatty meal
	Vyvanse and Adzenys	May want to take away from food	Food delays peak levels by 1 hour (Mydayis and the MR methylphenidates are not significantly affected by food)
	Valbenazine (Ingrezza)	Best to take away from a large meal	A high-fat meal lowers peak level by 50% and total serum levels by 10%
	Sildenafil (Viagra) and vardenafil (Levitra)	Best to take away from a high-fat meal (but alcohol has no effect); tadalafil (Cialis) and avanafil (Stendra) do not have food interactions	A high-fat meal lowers the peak by 20%–50% and delays the effects by 1 hour

by 25% when taken with food. Similarly, both ziprasidone (Geodon) and lurasidone (Latuda) are not absorbed very well unless they are taken with a meal. One explanatory theory regarding ziprasidone is that its capsules require extra acid to dissolve into absorbable form, and what better way to provide that acid than to stimulate its production with food?

Food effects vary by patient as well as by the food consumed. The phosphodiesterase (PDE5) inhibitors sildenafil (Viagra) and vardenafil (Levitra) are well-known examples of this effect. We have the most complete data for sildenafil, where a "high fat" meal delays absorption by an hour and reduces the eventual Tmax by 30%. Practical advice for patients? Stick with moderate-fat meals after taking the pill, or wait an hour or two after fatty meals. But if they *must* eat that extra-cheese pizza right away, having them take a higher-than-normal dose is reasonable, since this will at least ensure that an effective concentration will eventually be achieved.

Tables 13-1 and 13-2 list medications that are best absorbed with or without meals. To keep things simple, we've classified these food directions as *essential* or *optional*.

VERDICT

Get in the habit of writing "Take with a full meal" or "Take on an empty stomach" when prescribing medications with significant food interactions. If the patient doesn't follow those directions, you may need to raise or lower the dose to adjust for the effect. Keep these interactions in mind when taking a past history. For example, if a patient reports no benefit on lurasidone, ask if they remembered to take it with food.

Effects of Certain Drugs on Absorption

So far we have focused on how food changes medication absorption. But there are also some common drugs that can affect absorption of psychotropics. Antacids like Tums (calcium carbonate), Mylanta, and Maalox (combinations of magnesium and aluminum hydroxide) can enhance absorption of certain drugs such as diazepam (Valium) and ibuprofen. Other drugs slow down the stomach and impede gastric emptying, potentially decreasing drug absorption. The most common culprits are the opiate narcotics, including codeine, Percocet, Vicodin, and OxyContin. Patients on these meds might require higher doses of certain psych meds to achieve therapeutic levels.

Bioactive Foods: Grapefruit

Grapefruit raises the levels of several medications, including many psychiatric meds. The compounds in grapefruit that cause this interaction are furanocoumarins, and they are strong-to-moderate inhibitors of the enzyme CYP3A4. One grapefruit, or 2/3 of a cup of juice, is enough to make a difference, doubling or tripling the levels of victim medications. The effect is more pronounced within the first 6 hours after consumption and drops by 75% at 24 hours post-grapefruit.

This interaction is usually benign, but may cause problems with carbamazepine and certain benzos or antipsychotics (see following table). Older patients tend to eat more grapefruit, and they are also more prone to the adverse effects of higher medication levels, like sedation with the benzos or hypotension from antipsychotics.

VERDICT

When a patient has side effects on medications that are metabolized through CYP3A4, grapefruit may be part of the puzzle.

TABLE 13-3. Med Levels Raised by Grapefruit

Lumateperone (Caplyta), lurasidone (Latuda), pimavanserin (Nuplazid), quetiapine, ziprasidone (but not clozapine)
Carbamazepine
Clomipramine, fluvoxamine
Buspirone
Diazepam, temazepam, triazolam, quazepam
Suvorexant (Belsomra), lemborexant (Dayvigo)
Methadone, oxycodone
Oral esketamine (unknown if intranasal esketamine is affected)
Sildenafil, vardenafil, and tadalafil

Dose Dumping

Dose dumping is when the release mechanism in a modified-release (MR) formulation breaks down, causing the entire day's dosage to be released at once. Alcohol and fatty meals have this effect on some medications. There are three situations where you need to know about dose dumping:

1. **Quetiapine XR (Seroquel XR).** Dose dumping is such a problem with quetiapine XR that the prescribing information warns against taking it within an hour of a meal that is more than 300 calories.

2. **Generic MR medications.** To manufacture a generic MR medication, the company has to reverse-engineer the complex details of the release mechanism. That has led to some quality control issues, including a notorious case of dose dumping that caused the FDA to pull the 300 mg size of Teva's generic Wellbutrin XL (Budeprion XL) from the market.

3. **Opioids.** Some patients intentionally combine alcohol with their controlled-release opioids to speed the opioids' release and enhance the high.

Not every MR medication is vulnerable to dose dumping. For example, food actually delays the absorption of Adderall XR, and to a lesser extent Adzenys and Vyvanse.

VERDICT

Advise patients to take quetiapine XR on an empty stomach (1 hour away from food) to avoid dose dumping. Outside of that, dose dumping is pretty rare in psychiatry, although it may crop up from time to time in generic MR formulations.

CHAPTER 14

Recreational Drug Interactions

NEARLY EVERY PSYCHIATRIC MEDICATION HAS a cautionary note in its FDA labeling about combining it with alcohol or recreational drugs. Psychiatric medications are rarely tested with recreational drugs, so with a few exceptions these risks are theoretical. Unfortunately, these warnings are more likely to cause people to stop their psych meds than to give up their drug of abuse.

And that would be a bad thing. Antipsychotics and mood stabilizers may protect patients against a number of adverse reactions to drugs of abuse, including mania, psychosis, seizures, and neurotoxicity. In those cases, advise your patient that the drug they are abusing is unsafe on its own terms, but is even more unsafe without the medication on board. Exceptions do exist where recreational drugs can have serious interactions with psychiatric medications, and we'll discuss them in this chapter.

Smoking

Nicotine does not have pharmacokinetic interactions with psychiatric medications, but smoke does. Whether from tobacco, marijuana, or cloves, smoke is an inducer of the CYP1A2 enzyme. Vaping and e-cigs do not significantly affect that enzyme because they lack the polycyclic aromatic hydrocarbons responsible for its induction.

Usually, induction takes a while to kick in, but smoking is an exception to this rule. It only takes about 3 days for cigarette smoke to become a clinically meaningful inducer, and the reversal of that induction only takes about a week. The strength of this interaction varies with the amount of smoking. It is less pronounced in the occasional marijuana smoker, but with pack-a-day cigarette smokers it can be potent.

While blood levels of various antipsychotics and antidepressants are reduced by smoking, the most clinically relevant interaction is with

TABLE 14-1. Potential Interactions Between Recreational Drugs and Psychiatric Medications

Recreational Drug	Psych Med	Result of Interaction
Alcohol, opioids	Benzos, sedatives, barbiturates	Respiratory depression and death
Alcohol with a high tyramine content	MAOIs	Hypertensive crisis
Alcohol	Flibanserin (Addyi)	Syncope
Alcohol	Disulfiram	Severe hangover symptoms and potential cardiac arrest, respiratory depression, or seizures
Cannabis and CBD oil	Various	Inhibition of CYP2D6 and 3A4
Cocaine, meth	MAOIs	Hypertensive crisis
Cocaine, meth	Stimulants	Psychosis, cardiac arrest
LSD, MDMA ("ecstasy"), cocaine, amphetamines	Serotonergic medication (SSRIs, SNRIs, MAOIs, clomipramine, lithium)	Serotonin syndrome; SSRIs may reduce the euphoric effects of MDMA
LSD	Serotonergic medication (SSRIs, SNRIs, MAOIs, clomipramine, lithium)	Activation of hallucinogen-persisting perception disorder (this is when former LSD users have mild illusions of colors and shapes)
Opioids	Naltrexone	Naltrexone causes acute opioid withdrawal and should not be started until free of opioids for 1 week
Smoking	Various (see Table 14-2)	Induction of CYP1A2

clozapine and olanzapine—in both cases, serum levels decrease by up to 50%. If the patient suddenly stops smoking, the serum levels will rise. That can be a problem when psychotic patients are admitted to smoke-free inpatient units. If you admit a patient on clozapine who is forced to stop smoking, you should gradually decrease the dose by about 10% per day for 5 days to avoid worsening side effects (Demler TL, *US Pharm* 2012;37(11):HS16–HS19).

VERDICT

Be aware of the potential effects of "reversal of induction" when patients on antipsychotics stop smoking. Depending on their antipsychotic, levels may rise significantly.

**TABLE 14-2. Interactions Between Smoking
and Psychiatric Medications**

Smoking Tobacco or Marijuana Can Lower the Following	
Antipsychotics	Clozapine, haloperidol, olanzapine
Antidepressants	Duloxetine, fluvoxamine, mirtazapine
Other	Caffeine, propranolol, ramelteon

Note: Vaping and e-cigs do not cause this interaction

Alcohol and Acetaldehyde

Alcohol is the only psychoactive drug we know of that doesn't have a half-life. That means it leaves the body at a linear rate, as opposed to the exponential rate of medications that exit by halves. No matter how much a person drinks, the body can only clear alcohol at a steady rate of 3 mL per hour. There's an evolutionary advantage to this metabolic curiosity. Alcohol is metabolized to a poisonous compound: acetaldehyde. To protect us from toxic acetaldehyde levels, the liver has to wait for this poison to clear before it can metabolize more alcohol.

That protection only goes so far, as anyone who has woken up with a hangover knows. Acetaldehyde is responsible for most of the fatigue, headaches, and nausea that come with hangovers. It's also toxic at the cellular level, which contributes to many of the health risks associated with alcohol: hepatitis, heart disease, and cancer.

Disulfiram (Antabuse) works by blocking the enzyme that metabolizes acetaldehyde: acetaldehyde dehydrogenase. The result is that the body can't get rid of acetaldehyde, and one sip of alcohol will cause an immediate hangover effect from the acetaldehyde buildup. Too many drinks can be fatal. Patients need to be sober for at least 12 hours before starting disulfiram, and its effects on alcohol metabolism can last up to 2 weeks after the last dose.

Some antibiotics have disulfiram-like effects on alcohol metabolism, most notably metronidazole, ketoconazole, and griseofulvin.

Cocaine, Opioids, CBD Oil, and More

There are a few situations where recreational drugs can cause serious problems when taken with psychiatric medications. Benzodiazepines and opioids are both respiratory suppressants, and their combined use is responsible for many of the accidental deaths in the opioid epidemic. This is also true for opioid replacement therapies like methadone, and to a lesser extent buprenorphine/naloxone (Suboxone).

An important drug interaction related to methadone is the induction of its metabolism by carbamazepine. Patients on methadone maintenance who are also on carbamazepine may require heroic doses of methadone to stave off dope-sickness—for example, in the range of 180–240 mg daily. If such a patient then takes a CYP3A4 inhibitor, they may experience dangerous methadone toxicity such as QTc prolongation. The bottom line? Prescribe carbamazepine to methadone users with caution.

Psychostimulants can lead to cardiac arrest when taken with cocaine or other amphetamines. Multiple recreational drugs can cause serotonin syndrome or a hypertensive crisis when taken with MAOIs or serotonergic antidepressants (see Table 14-1). Kratom (*Mitragyna speciosa*) is an emerging drug of abuse that is also likely to cause problems with MAOIs, as it has dopaminergic and serotonergic effects as well as opioid agonism. Kratom can also cause significant drug interactions as an inhibitor of CYP2D6, 3A4, and 1A2 enzymes. There has been one reported death after kratom use that was attributed to high levels of quetiapine, a 3A4 substrate.

Enzymatic inhibition is also a problem with CBD oil (cannabidiol). This extract of marijuana does not contain THC, which is responsible for marijuana's high (although THC may be present as an impurity in some products). CBD is not a drug of abuse, but patients are increasingly using it to relieve anxiety, sleep, or pain. Recent studies suggest that CBD may raise levels of psychiatric medications by inhibiting metabolic enzymes. So far, we have heard of inhibitory effects at CYP2D6, 3A4, 1A2, 2B6, 2C8, 2C9, 2C19, and 2E1, as well as UGT1A9 and UGT2B7. If these in vitro effects translate to human studies, the effects we'd be most concerned with are toxicity on carbamazepine (3A4, 2C8) or tricyclic antidepressants (2D6, 2C19) and a higher risk of rash when titrating lamotrigine (UGT1A9) (Brown JD et al, *J Clin Med* 2019;8(7):989).

VERDICT

Warn patients about recreational drugs that have dangerous interactions with the psychiatric medications they are taking. Ask about CBD and kratom use, which may raise the levels and heighten the side effects of many psychotropics.

CHAPTER 15

Pharmacodynamic Drug Interactions

PHARMACOKINETICS REFERS TO THE WAYS that the body affects a drug, mainly by altering its serum levels. Pharmaco*dynamics* is how a drug affects the body. In psychiatry, "the body" usually refers to the neurotransmitter systems in the brain, but drugs can interact with other organs as well. In this chapter, we'll focus on the most dangerous pharmacodynamic interactions in psychiatry:

1. Respiratory suppression from benzodiazepines taken with opioids
2. Hypertensive crisis from monoamine oxidase inhibitors (MAOI) interacting with various medications and foods
3. Serotonin syndrome from the additive effects of various medications
4. Anticholinergic side effects
5. Cardiac arrhythmias from drugs that prolong the QTc interval

Opioids and Benzodiazepines

When the benzodiazepines were first released in 1960, they were welcomed as a safer alternative to the barbiturates, which were causing a rash of overdose deaths at the time. For several decades, the benzos lived up to this promise; very few people died from them. Then came the expansion of opioids in the 1990s, and now we are living with a new problem caused by a pharmacodynamic interaction between these two drugs.

The problem is that benzodiazepines and opioids both suppress breathing, but they do so in different ways. Opioids act in the medulla, while benzos turn down respiratory drive through $GABA_A$ inhibition. The effect is much like a stereo system: Unplug one speaker and you can still hear the music, but unplug both and breathing stops. Alcohol can add to the problem, as it suppresses respiration much like benzodiazepines do.

135

TABLE 15-1. When to Avoid Benzos in Patients on Opioids

Near-absolute contraindication	• Active prescription misuse • Active addiction to benzos, opioids, alcohol, or other sedatives • History of sedative overdose • Methadone use
Strong relative contraindication	• History of sedative, alcohol, or opioid use disorder • Borderline or antisocial personality disorder • Unstable psychiatric disorder • Respiratory disease (eg, COPD, sleep apnea), systemic medical illness (eg, HIV, organ failure, renal or hepatic impairment), or pregnancy • Daily opioid dose ≥ 50 morphine milligram equivalents (see www.oregonpainguidance.org/opioidmedcalculator); long-acting opioids carry a higher risk than short-acting ones • Age ≥ 65

Just how much do benzodiazepines raise the risk of opioid-related fatalities? About 2- to 4-fold, according to a study of over 100,000 veterans that controlled for confounding variables (Park TW et al, *BMJ* 2015;350:h2698). Many of these deaths were accidental and did not involve substance abuse or suicidal intent.

As medical boards have cracked down on benzo-opioid polypharmacy, other physicians are referring patients on both drugs to psychiatrists to take over the benzodiazepine script. Here's how to handle those challenging referrals (see Table 15-1). Essentially, you should avoid prescribing benzos to any patient who is actively overusing sedatives or who has a history of sedative overdose. Next, figure out how necessary the benzodiazepine actually is. The clearest indication for its use is panic disorder, with generalized anxiety and social anxiety disorders a close second. Without a clearly diagnosed anxiety disorder, long-term use of a benzodiazepine is harder to justify.

Patients in the "near-absolute contraindication" category (see Table 15-1) will usually need to stop either the benzo, the opioid, or both. For those at lower risk levels, it's still a good idea to attempt to taper off the benzo or replace it with another therapy. Successful benzodiazepine tapering strategies are usually very gradual and include plenty of support beyond the tapering itself. If that is unsuccessful, try switching to a benzodiazepine with a lower risk of overdose. The risk is higher with rapid-acting, highly rewarding benzos (especially clonazepam, alprazolam, and diazepam). The lowest risk is with oxazepam, which takes 1–2 hours to take effect (as opposed to 30 minutes for most other benzos). Oxazepam also leaves the body quickly, further lowering the likelihood of an interaction. Lorazepam is a close second to oxazepam in terms of overdose risk (Buckley NA et al, *BMJ* 1995;310(6974):219–221).

MAOIs, Cheese, and the Hypertensive Crisis

Perhaps the most dreaded side effect in psychiatry is the interaction of MAOIs with tyramine-rich foods like cheese, which can cause a hypertensive crisis. This is a sharp and severe spike in blood pressure, typically to levels beyond 180/120 mmHg.

While everyday hypertension is a "silent killer," slowly damaging the body without causing the patient any symptoms, hypertensive crises are not silent. The vascular system has no time to adjust to the sudden increase in blood pressure. Vessels can burst, causing end-organ damage and stroke. Signs of hypertensive crisis include severe headache, confusion, blurry vision, chest pain, and seizures.

The MAOI-Cheese Interaction: Some Historical Perspective

In the first few years after MAOIs were introduced, nobody had an inkling of their potential dietary interactions. Then in 1961, a case report was published in *The Lancet* of a woman who died of a subarachnoid hemorrhage while taking tranylcypromine (Parnate), but clinicians were slow to blame tranylcypromine because these events occurred often enough in patients who were not taking MAOIs.

It took a psychiatric resident to save the day. Barry Blackwell, who was training at the Maudsley Hospital in London at the time, began reading about sporadic cases of high blood pressure, headache, and subarachnoid hemorrhage in patients taking MAOIs. A pharmacist told Blackwell that the pharmacist's wife, who was taking an MAOI, had developed two episodes of hypertension and headache after eating cheese. Intrigued, Blackwell and a colleague experimented on themselves. They took tranylcypromine for a week, then gorged on cheese. They felt perfectly fine. Nonetheless, in his hospital, Blackwell consulted on several cases where patients taking MAOIs developed hypertensive headaches after eating cheese sandwiches. He published his suspicions in *Lancet* in 1963, but it still took some time before a skeptical medical community took this MAOI-cheese connection seriously, partly because there was no known mechanism to explain it. (For more details and references related to this story, see the fascinating book *The Antidepressant Era* by David Healy, Harvard University Press, 1997.)

This historical aside is interesting because it affords some perspective on the dangers of MAOI interactions. MAOIs were prescribed frequently for several years by physicians who had no knowledge of their possible drug or food interactions, and yet the rate of fatal reactions was extremely low. With our current knowledge of these interactions, the risk of serious problems is even lower.

The MAOI-Tyramine Interaction Explained

MAOIs, as their name implies, inactivate the enzyme monoamine oxidase (MAO). This MAO enzyme comes in two forms: A and B. MAO-A is the troublesome molecule in this story, because its normal function is to metabolize and break down the neurotransmitters serotonin, norepinephrine, and to some extent dopamine. Thus, tranylcypromine, phenelzine, and isocarboxazid increase levels of all three of these neurotransmitters by inhibiting MAO-A.

These changes in neurotransmitter levels ease symptoms of both depression and anxiety, and MAOI side effects are generally fairly tolerable: insomnia or sedation, orthostatic dizziness, lowered libido, and occasional weight gain. When no dangerous interactions enter the equation, MAOIs are tolerated better than tricyclic antidepressants and a bit worse than selective serotonin reuptake inhibitors (SSRIs), and they are considered by some authorities to be more effective than either tricyclics or SSRIs for depression with atypical features (overeating, oversleeping, and leaden paralysis).

Enter cheese. Certain cheeses, in addition to several other foods and beverages, contain high quantities of the amino acid tyramine. Why is tyramine potentially hazardous? To answer that, it's helpful to know that tyramine is produced from another amino acid, tyrosine. Tyrosine is (or should be) quite famous among psychiatrists, because it is the precursor of both dopamine and norepinephrine. To return to biochemistry class for a minute, the synthetic pathway is:

$$Tyrosine \rightarrow DOPA \rightarrow Dopamine \rightarrow Norepinephrine$$

The action of norepinephrine is terminated by the enzyme MAO-A, as well as by another enzyme, catechol-O-methyl-transferase. By a separate pathway, tyrosine can also be transformed to tyramine, which, like norepinephrine, is broken down by MAO-A. At this point, you might be thinking that because MAOIs prevent tyramine's breakdown, this leads to a buildup of tyramine's precursor, tyrosine, leading to too much dopamine and norepinephrine via the synthetic pathway outlined above. While this roundabout mechanism is part of the story, the major way that excess tyramine causes high blood pressure is via a more immediate effect on norepinephrine.

Tyramine is sometimes termed a false neurotransmitter because it gets actively transported into neurons and displaces norepinephrine, increasing norepinephrine levels in the bloodstream (Meck JV et al, *J Cardiovasc Pharmacol* 2003;41(1):126–131). This, in turn, can result in vasoconstriction and hypertension. In fact, when volunteers who are not taking MAOIs ingest large amounts of tyramine, they experience a small rise in blood pressure, because it takes a little while for the body's MAO enzymes to metabolize this extra tyramine (VanDenBerg CM et al, *J Clin Pharmacol* 2003;43(6):604–609).

Now imagine dumping tyramine into a body that does not have any functioning MAO enzymes, as would be the situation for a patient on MAOIs. In this case, there is a double whammy of norepinephrine. First, the MAOI inhibits the breakdown of norepinephrine directly; second, the tyramine, acting as an independent false neurotransmitter, displaces norepinephrine from nerve terminals (see Figure 15-1). The combined effect floods the body with norepinephrine, causing vasoconstriction, severe hypertension, and potentially catastrophic sequelae like stroke.

EMSAM: A Safer MAOI?

Selegiline is an MAOI that we use for depression as the EMSAM patch, but it began its life as an oral medication for Parkinson's disease. Unlike traditional MAOIs, which inhibit the MAO-A receptor, selegiline is selective

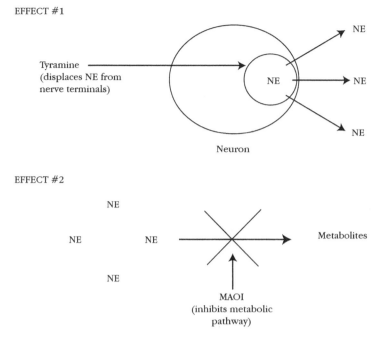

FIGURE 15-1. "Double Whammy" Effect of Ingesting Tyramine With MAOI on Board

for MAO-B. This receptor is not involved in depression, so oral selegiline's antidepressant effects don't kick in until the dose gets high enough for its inhibitor effects to spread to MAO-A (around 30 mg/day of oral selegiline). At that dose, it also inhibits MAO-A in the gut and requires the same dietary precautions as traditional MAOIs.

Transdermal selegiline (EMSAM) was developed to get around this problem. The medication passes directly into the bloodstream through the skin, bypassing the liver and GI tract. This, in turn, yields two metabolic benefits. First, because transdermal selegiline's concentration in the GI tract is much lower than the oral version, there is less inhibition of dietary tyramine's metabolism, and so less concern about dietary restrictions. Second, because there is no first-pass effect through the liver, a relatively low amount of selegiline can provide therapeutic concentrations in the brain, minimizing systemic side effects (9 mg/day of transdermal selegiline equates to 30 mg/day of oral selegiline).

What all this means is that EMSAM does not require any dietary restrictions, but this is true only at the starting dose of 6 mg/day. At the higher doses of 9 and 12 mg/day, all the usual restrictions apply, because at these doses enough of the medication gets into the gut to inhibit the metabolism of tyramine. However, if you take a look at the raw data used by the FDA to make these crucial dosing decisions, you come away with the sense that they were extremely cautious, and that in fact the 9 mg dose is likely to be quite safe without dietary restrictions. In clinical practice, this means you can be somewhat less insistent that patients follow their MAOI diet when they are on EMSAM 9 mg than if they are on the highest dose, 12 mg.

To increase the confusion, the entire discussion above applies only to MAOI food interactions and not MAOI drug interactions. EMSAM is considered dangerous to combine with serotonergic drugs at *all* doses, including the 6 mg dose. This is because these drug interactions have nothing to do with tyramine and generally involve excessive serotonin. However, since EMSAM was released, there have been many cases of patients taking supposedly forbidden medications without suffering serotonin syndrome. (For a comprehensive review of EMSAM's safety record, see Asnis G and Henderson M, *Neuropsychiatr Dis Treat* 2014;10:1911–1923.)

So, is EMSAM a safer MAOI? Probably so, and as we gain more experience using it, we'll all likely become more comfortable with it, which is a good thing for those patients who have failed all the usual antidepressant suspects.

Tyramine in the Diet

How do foods get to be high in tyramine? Through the action of bacteria on tyrosine, which high-protein foods have lots of. Bacteria such as *Enterococcus* and *Lactobacillus* contain tyrosine decarboxylase, which converts tyrosine to tyramine. Hence, foods that contain amino acids (eg, have protein) and have a lot of bacteria in them are likely to be loaded with tyramine. One of the best ways for bacteria to grow is by allowing food to sit around for a long time, which is why aged foods of all sorts are on the high tyramine list: stinky cheeses, smoked meats, and fermented liquids (beer, certain wines, soy sauce). This is also why we tell patients on MAOIs to eat foods when they are fresh. The longer cheese or meat is left in the fridge, the more bacteria, and hence the more tyramine.

The internet is awash with lists of foods to avoid with MAOIs, but most of those are out of date. It's only in the past two decades that we've had the technology to accurately measure tyramine in food. Since then, the restrictions have relaxed a bit, most importantly with pizza. Researchers at the University of Toronto found that pizzas from major food chains had safe quantities of tyramine, including a Domino's double-cheese, double-pepperoni pizza (Shulman KI and Walker SE, *J Clin Psychiatry* 1999;60(3):191–193). The serving sizes were liberal: half of a medium pizza.

TABLE 15-2. A Modernized MAOI Diet

Avoid completely	Highly aged cheeses and aged beef (eg, charcuterie boards) Freshly baked sourdough bread Fermented soy bean products (found in Asian foods like tempeh, miso, pickled tofu, and bean paste) Fermented meat or fish Raw meat or fish that has not been refrigerated properly or is past its use-by date Homemade beer or wine
OK in small portions (less than a typical serving size)	Specialty soy sauce Dried, aged sausage and salami (prosciutto is OK) Sauerkraut Beer that is microbrewed, on tap, or requires refrigeration (no more than 1 standard drink)
OK in normal portions (but don't overindulge)	Cheeses that are not highly aged Chocolate Caffeinated beverages Wine from a commercial producer (no more than 2 glasses) Beer that is shelf-stable or pasteurized (no more than 2 pints) Fresh beef or fish Fava beans Bananas and avocados that aren't overly ripe Soy sauce or fish sauce from grocery store brands Worcestershire sauce Kimchi Commercially produced sourdough bread Fermented yeast products (Marmite and Vegemite)
No restrictions (barely any tyramine here)	Milk, yogurt, cream Non-matured, soft cheese (mozzarella, American, ricotta, cottage cheese, cream cheese) Dry, cured meats (prosciutto, pepperoni) Smoked or pickled fish Fresh chicken, duck, pork, and sausage Stock cubes, powder, or bullion Non-fermented soy bean products

Sources: psychotropical.com; Finberg JPM and Gillman K, *Int Rev Neurobiol* 2011;100:169–190

MAOIs, SSRIs, and Serotonin Syndrome

The tyramine "cheese" effect may be the most famous and feared MAOI interaction, but serotonin syndrome is probably more common and can be just as serious. In fact, the most infamous case involving MAOIs, the Libby Zion case, involved a death due to serotonin syndrome in which an MAOI was combined with the serotonergic opioid meperidine, causing malignant hyperthermia and death from cardiac arrest. The resident who prescribed this combination to Zion had been awake for 18 hours, and it was this case that set in motion the restrictions in on-call hours that residents (and patients) now benefit from.

Serotonin syndrome is best thought of as serotonin toxicity, and it occurs on a spectrum, from barely recognizable to potentially lethal. At the mild level are serotonergic side effects like jitteriness, insomnia, GI disturbances, and cognitive problems like word-finding difficulties or general spaciness. As these serotonergic effects become more extreme, they eventually cross a line and become the serotonin syndrome. Think of "shaking, sweaty, and confused" to remember its hallmark symptoms:

- Shaking: muscle jerking (myoclonus), tremor, akathisia
- Sweaty: fever, sweating
- Confused: mental status changes, delirium

Of all these symptoms, the most reliable for accurately diagnosing serotonin syndrome are the neuromuscular symptoms, such as myoclonus (rapid alternating relaxation and contraction of muscles, often measured by flexing the patient's foot and watching for rhythmic contractions of the ankle), hyperreflexia, and muscular rigidity. These can help differentiate it from neuroleptic malignant syndrome (NMS), a rare reaction to antipsychotics. Both syndromes can present with autonomic instability, mental status changes, and rigidity, but unlike NMS, serotonin syndrome is rapidly progressive and includes hyperreflexia in addition to the rigidity.

A Controversial Issue: How Relevant Is Serotonin Syndrome in Clinical Practice?

While there is no disagreement in the field about the fact that serotonin syndrome exists and can be deadly, there is much controversy about how common it is and which drug combinations cause it. As with any controversial topic in medicine, there are different factions arguing their points. The inclusive faction argues that serotonin syndrome is more common and less predictable than appreciated, while the purist faction argues that the syndrome occurs primarily in clear situations of serotonin toxicity.

In the next section, we'll take a hard-nosed look at which medication combinations are most likely to lead to serotonin syndrome.

Specific Drug Combinations: An Evaluation of the Dangers

Serotonin syndrome can occur from an overdose of serotonergic medication or from a drug interaction between two serotonergics. Although SSRIs are prone to this interaction, it is with MAOIs that serotonin syndrome is the most common and most dangerous. MAOIs increase serotonin by blocking the MAO-A enzyme. When used on their own, this effect is therapeutic. But when another serotonergic medication is added in, the body is unable to break down the excess serotonin, resulting in toxicity.

The risk of this interaction is illustrated by a large database of 2222 cases of serotonergic drug overdose in the Newcastle region of Australia from 1987 to 2002. Overdoses on an SSRI led to serotonin syndrome 15% of the time, but when the overdose involved both an SSRI and MAOI, the rate of serotonin syndrome rose to 50%. The cases involving MAOIs were also much more severe (Dunkley EJC et al, *QJM* 2003;96(9):635–642).

That same Australian group also gathered a practical list of medications you should avoid with MAOIs, and we've updated and reprinted that information in Table 15-3. Most of these medications can also cause serotonin syndrome when combined with SSRIs, but there the risk is much lower than it is with MAOIs. In the case of the sympathomimetics, which include psychostimulants, phentermine, and cocaine, combination with MAOIs risks not only serotonin syndrome but also hypertensive crisis.

Besides the usual round of antidepressants, we should also watch out for ziprasidone, the lone antipsychotic that can't be taken with an MAOI. Ziprasidone is a serotonin 1A agonist with a track record for triggering serotonin syndrome in case reports. In addition to psychiatric medications, the list includes a few opioids with serotonergic properties. Morphine, codeine, oxycodone, and buprenorphine (the active ingredient in Suboxone) are safe. There are also a few over-the-counter medications to warn patients about.

TABLE 15-3. Medications That Can Cause Serotonin Syndrome With MAOIs*

Serotonergic psychotropics	Serotonergic antidepressants (SSRIs, SNRIs, other MAOIs, vortioxetine, vilazodone, clomipramine, imipramine, and possibly trazodone and nefazodone); ketamine, esketamine, viloxazine, ziprasidone, and possibly lithium and buspirone
Stimulants	Amphetamine, methylphenidate, phentermine, and local anesthetics that contain sympathomimetics
Serotonergic opioids	Fentanyl, methadone, meperidine, oxycodone, propoxyphene, tramadol
Other	Fenfluramine, linezolid, methylene blue, moclobemide
Over-the-counter	L-tryptophan, SAMe, St. John's wort, and decongestants containing phenylephrine, pseudoephedrine, dextromethorphan, or chlorpheniramine
Drugs of abuse	Cocaine, amphetamines, LSD, MDMA, ecstasy, bath salts

*These meds can also cause serotonin syndrome with SSRIs and SNRIs, but the risk with these combinations is much lower

One of them—pseudoephedrine—is now kept behind the counter to prevent diversion into meth labs, but it is still available without a prescription.

The savvy reader may also notice a few medications that are missing from the list. Some medicines were thought to cause serotonin syndrome on theoretical grounds, but those concerns did not hold up over time. For example, the triptans treat migraines by activating serotonin 1B and 1D receptors. Those receptors are not implicated in serotonin syndrome, and a database of over 19,000 patients who took triptans with serotonergic antidepressants also failed to implicate them (Orlova Y et al, *JAMA Neurol* 2018;75(5):566–572). Although triptans' association with serotonin syndrome is increasingly in doubt, it's worth knowing that the following triptans are considered safest: almotriptan (Axert), naratriptan (Amerge), eletriptan (Relpax), and frovatriptan (Frova).

Carbamazepine is another medication we gave a pass to. This anticonvulsant has a structural resemblance to the tricyclic antidepressants, which generated concerns that it might interact with MAOIs, but those suspicions have not panned out. Also missing from our list are the alpha-antagonists like clonidine and guanfacine, which appear on some "do not combine with MAOIs" lists. We left them off because here the risk is not serotonin syndrome but orthostatic hypotension, a common problem with MAOIs that antihypertensives can exacerbate.

Controversy: Antidepressant Augmentation of MAOIs

Combining a serotonergic antidepressant with an MAOI is potentially lethal, but what about adding a non-serotonergic antidepressant? This strategy is controversial, but as reassuring case series have built up over the years it has become slightly more acceptable. Among the tricyclic antidepressants, the noradrenergic tricyclics (desipramine, trimipramine, and doxepin) are probably safe, but the serotonergic tricyclics should be avoided (imipramine and—the most serotonergic of all—clomipramine). Bupropion, mirtazapine, and trazodone (which has been used successfully to treat MAOI-induced insomnia) are all relatively low risk.

Another risky strategy is combining psychostimulants with MAOIs, which can cause both serotonin syndrome and a hypertensive crisis. However, both of these problems are fairly rare, with only a few case reports in the past 50 years. Some experts utilize this combination in refractory depression to create a "triple reuptake inhibitor" that raises serotonin, norepinephrine, and dopamine. Among the two stimulants, methylphenidate is safer to combine with MAOIs than the amphetamines. The risk is further reduced by adding stimulants to MAOIs slowly and at low doses.

While these MAOI combination strategies may be appropriate for patients with severe, refractory depression in the hands of careful, experienced clinicians, they're not for everyday use. At the very least, monitor blood pressure when embarking on them.

Switching to and From MAOIs

To prevent serotonin syndrome, a washout period is required between stopping a serotonergic drug and replacing it with an MAOI. Once the old drug is completely stopped, wait at least 5–7 half-lives for it to clear before starting the MAOI. Technically, 5 half-lives should be enough, but there may still be some residual reuptake inhibition after all the actual medication has washed out of the patient's system. For most antidepressants that means waiting 1–2 weeks, for fluoxetine the wait is 4–5 weeks, and for vortioxetine it's 2–3 weeks. Patients will worry about going that long without an antidepressant, but reassure them that the drug is still in their system and use benzodiazepines if any serious distress arises during the washout (alprazolam, in particular, had rapid effects against depression in over a dozen controlled trials).

When switching from any MAOI to a serotonergic medication, wait 14 days before starting the new medication. Because most MAOIs have a half-life of 24 hours (or less), a 14-day washout is conservative. That time period takes into account the fact that currently available MAOIs are *irreversible* inhibitors of MAO, meaning that the enzyme is essentially destroyed. After the drug is gone, the body needs another week or so to remanufacture enough MAO in order to safely deal with the SSRI/SNRI. This same rule applies when switching from one MAOI to another.

TABLE 15-4. The Human Cost of Anticholinergic Drugs

Anticholinergic Effect	Why It Matters
Dry mouth	Tooth decay, gum inflammation and ulceration; poor dental hygiene is a risk factor for depression and dementia
Constipation	Bowel obstruction with potentially fatal paralytic ileus and sepsis
Urinary retention	Urinary tract infections, renal or bladder damage
Dilated pupils	Acute narrow-angle glaucoma, traffic accidents, falls
Impaired papillary accommodation	Inability to read fine print
Increased heart rate	Increased risk of cardiac arrest
Decreased sweating	Hyperthermia
Decreased bronchial secretions	Mucous plugging of small airways, which worsens respiratory illnesses like asthma and bronchitis
Cognitive impairment	Poor memory and concentration; delirium; increased risk of dementia

Anticholinergic Burden

There are two sides of the autonomic nervous system: the sympathetic system and the parasympathetic system. The parasympathetic system manages physiological activities during rest, so it is sometimes called the "rest and digest" system. It relies on the neurotransmitter acetylcholine, the effects of which are often summarized with the mnemonic "SLUD": Salivation, Lacrimation, Urination, Defecation. In other words, acetylcholine causes drooling and tearing up of the eyes, and facilitates both

TABLE 15-5. Anticholinergic Burden

	Very Low (0)	Low (1)	Medium (2)	High (3)
Antidepressants		Bupropion Citalopram Fluoxetine Fluvoxamine Selegiline Trazodone Venlafaxine	Desipramine Sertraline Trimipramine	Amitriptyline Clomipramine Doxepin Imipramine Nortriptyline Paroxetine
Antipsychotics	Brexpiprazole Lumateperone Lurasidone Thiothixene Ziprasidone	Aripiprazole Asenapine Haloperidol Iloperidone Paliperidone Quetiapine Risperidone	Loxapine Pimozide Prochlorperazine	Amoxapine Chlorpromazine Clozapine Fluphenazine Olanzapine Perphenazine Thioridazine
Other		Alprazolam Clorazepate Diazepam Pramipexole	Amantadine Carbamazepine Oxcarbazepine	Benztropine Diphenhydramine Doxylamine (Unisom) Hydroxyzine

Source: www.acbcalc.com

urination and defecation. It's also involved in cognitive function, which is why many of our antidementia drugs inhibit the enzyme that breaks down acetylcholine.

Anticholinergic medications do the opposite of SLUD. They cause dry mouth, dry eyes (and blurry vision), urinary retention, constipation, and mental confusion. When those symptoms go on too long, they lead to more serious problems that are listed in Table 15-4, like bowel obstruction and tooth decay. There is also some evidence that they can increase the risk of dementia.

The key thing to remember as you treat patients is that combining drugs with anticholinergic properties can cause significant problems, especially in the elderly, who are prone to developing confusion and other side effects when overdosed on these drugs. Also be on the lookout for patients with schizophrenia. These patients have a hard time conveying their physical symptoms, and they often take a lot of anticholinergic medications. In 2020 the FDA issued a specific warning about combining clozapine with anticholinergics because they increase the risk of intestinal ileus, a potentially fatal form of constipation, 6-fold.

Anticholinergic effects are additive, so this is usually a problem of poly-pharmacy. The Anticholinergic Burden (ACB) score helps you gauge the problem as the medications stack up. Each medication is assigned a score of 1–3, where 1 represents possible anticholinergic effects (demonstrated in the lab but clinical effect is uncertain), 2 represents known anticholinergic effects, and 3 represents significant clinical effects (eg, can cause delirium).

We've listed the psychiatric culprits in Table 15-5, along with some good alternatives that have very low risks, but it's worthwhile to check the patient's full regimen at www.acbcalc.com. The full list includes over 150 medications and was last updated in 2012.

Here's how you might use the ACB score in practice. In terms of toler-ability, younger patients probably won't notice much until the score gets to 3. Patients over age 50 might experience problems at a score of 2, and these may become more serious after age 65. The scale has also been used to predict long-term outcomes. Higher numbers predict falls, cognitive decline, and overall mortality, but the studies that found these associations were not randomized so they do not prove causation.

The QTc Burden

Another area where polypharmacy can turn a mild side effect into a major problem is prolongation of the QTc interval. This is the interval between the Q and T waves on an EKG, which represents the time it takes for the ventricles to depolarize and repolarize. The QT interval varies with the heart rate, and the "c" in QTc means the measure is corrected for the heart rate. Normal QTc intervals are generally defined as < 460 msec for women and < 450 msec for men. QTc prolongation can lead to serious arrhythmias, including the potentially fatal torsades de pointes, particularly when the QTc rises above 500 msec.

Many medications can prolong the QTc, and the risk is greater at higher doses or when multiple QTc-prolonging agents are stacked together. A few psychotropics have specific warnings to avoid high doses—and drug interactions that can raise the dose—because of this danger (eg, citalopram, pimozide, thioridazine, deutetrabenazine, and valbenazine). However, reflexively lowering those doses can have unintended consequences. When the Veterans Administration lowered citalopram in 38,548 patients who were on a high dose of the antidepressant before the FDA warning, the risk of hospitalization and death went up 4-fold after the dose was lowered (Rector TS et al, *Am J Psychiatry* 2016;173(9):896–902).

Another controversy around the QTc is that this measure is only moderately associated with the outcome in question—torsades de pointes. Some drugs that have a high risk of prolonging the QTc, like ziprasidone, have a low risk of causing torsades de pointes. Part of the reason is that QTc is the sum of the depolarization and repolarization times, and it is only when the repolarization is prolonged that trouble starts to happen (and unfortunately, an EKG won't isolate the repolarization time).

The bottom line is that you can't judge the cardiac risk by the QTc alone. In the following table, we've grouped medications based on how likely they are to cause torsades de pointes, rather than prolong the QTc, based on rankings from Credible Meds (www.crediblemeds.org).

A few patterns stand out:

1. All antipsychotics carry a risk, but some are worse than others (eg, chlorpromazine, thioridazine), and older atypicals have a lower risk than the newer ones. Aripiprazole has the lowest risk of QTc prolongation, but is somewhere in the middle when it comes to the risk of torsades de pointes. Three treatments for tardive dyskinesia made the list, and these are often added to antipsychotics.

2. Among the SSRIs, escitalopram and especially citalopram have the highest risk, which is unfortunate because these are often favored in the elderly for their relative lack of drug interactions. Sertraline's risk is low, and this SSRI is also considered the safest for patients with cardiac disease. Tricyclics as a class have a high risk.

3. Three medications for dementia (memantine, donepezil, and galantamine) are on the list. These medications are often held up as candidates for deprescribing in the elderly because their meager benefits are often outweighed by their risks.

4. Only one medication for erectile dysfunction made the list: vardenafil (Levitra). Cross-checking with the *PDR* reveals that tadalafil (Cialis) has a minimal effect on QTc (about a third of vardenafil's), while sildenafil (Viagra) has no effect.

5. All of the ADHD medications pose risks in congenital long QT except the modafinils and alpha-2 agonists. Congenital long QT is a rare (1 in 2,500) genetic syndrome that puts patients at risk for sudden cardiac death with certain medications. Most experts do not recommend routine screening

TABLE 15-6. Risk of Torsades de Pointes With Psychiatric Medications

	Conditional (Low) Torsades Risk	Possible Torsades Risk	Known Torsades Risk	Only Dangerous in Congenital Long QT
Antidepressants	Amitriptyline Clomipramine Doxepin Fluoxetine Fluvoxamine Paroxetine Sertraline Trazodone	Desipramine Imipramine Maprotiline Mirtazapine Nortriptyline Trimipramine Venlafaxine	Citalopram Escitalopram	
Antipsychotics	Olanzapine Quetiapine Risperidone Ziprasidone	Aripiprazole Asenapine Clozapine Iloperidone Lumateperone Lurasidone Perphenazine Paliperidone Pimavanserin Promethazine	Chlorpromazine Haloperidol Pimozide Thioridazine	
ADHD		Atomoxetine		Psychostimulants
Other	Amantadine Chloral hydrate Diphenhydramine Galantamine Hydroxyzine	Buprenorphine Deutetrabenazine Dextromethorphan/ quinidine Lithium Memantine Pitolisant Tetrabenazine Valbenazine Vardenafil	Donepezil Methadone Ondansetron	

Source: www.crediblemeds.org

with EKGs for this syndrome because EKGs aren't sensitive or specific enough to pick up on the problem. Instead, these screening questions can help identify patients at risk for congenital long QT:

- Have you ever fainted or passed out during or after exercise, emotion, or startle?
- Have you ever had significant pain or pressure in your chest during exercise or felt your heart "racing" or "skipping beats" during exercise?

- Have any of your family members (blood relatives) died suddenly before the age of 30?

Outside of congenital long QT, there are also risk factors for torsades de pointes that would make us think twice before adding medications with known risks of torsades. The big three are low potassium, low magnesium, and heart disease (specifically, low left ventricular ejection fraction, left ventricular hypertrophy, ischemia, and slow heart rate). Other risks include older age, female gender, and recreational use of cocaine or stimulants.

Here's how to interpret the information in Table 15-6. Meds listed in "Conditional (Low) Torsades Risk" may cause torsades de pointes only in rare instances such as in overdose. Drugs in the "Possible Torsades Risk" column are not associated with torsades de pointes at normal doses but can prolong the QTc. The medications listed under "Known Torsades Risk" prolong the QTc and have been known to cause torsades de pointes even when taken on their own in normal doses. Finally, the items listed as "Only Dangerous in Congenital Long QT" are only known to cause problems in the 1 in 2,500 patients who are born with a long QTc. Note that for this population, the medications in all the other categories are also risky.

SECTION III

Special Topics

CHAPTER 16

Generic Medications and Drug Metabolism

GENERICS CONSTITUTE ABOUT 70% OF all prescriptions for psychotropics. Most medications in all categories of therapeutics are now available as generics, including stimulants, antidepressants, atypical antipsychotics, anxiolytics, and mood stabilizers.

The benefits of prescribing generic medications are clear—we reduce copayments for our patients and lower the overall financial burden on the health care system. But what about the potential disadvantages? Most psychiatrists have either had experience in their own practice or heard stories from colleagues about patients switched from brand to generic formulations who have had breakthrough psychiatric symptoms. The question is, aside from such anecdotal reports, is there scientific evidence documenting the bioequivalence of generics and brand-name medications in psychiatry?

We'll review the research on this topic, but first, it will be helpful to outline the history and current regulations of generics in the United States.

Generic Drugs: A Primer

The story of the modern generic drug industry began in 1984, when Congress passed the Hatch-Waxman Act in response to rising pharmaceutical costs. As we'll see, the act significantly loosened the requirements to get a generic medication approved by the FDA.

When a drug company discovers a new compound, it quickly applies for a series of patents, which last 20 years from the time the compound was first discovered. Of course, a good chunk of a compound's patent life is taken up with all the basic clinical research required to win FDA approval. Companies must first test drugs for safety in animals, then in human volunteers in Phase I trials, then in groups of patients in Phase II trials, and finally in very large groups of patients in Phase III trials. In order to receive FDA approval, companies must provide positive results of at least 2 large placebo-controlled trials. The drug testing and evaluation process takes an average of 10 years, so most drugs have only another 10 years of patent protection remaining after FDA approval. Nonetheless, a blockbuster drug can earn billions of dollars in that time span. (See the FDA's Office of Generic Drugs website at https://www.fda.gov/about-fda/center-drug-evaluation-and-research-cder/office-generic-drugs for more extensive information.)

Before the Hatch-Waxman Act, generic companies were required to go through the same time-consuming R&D process as the "originator" companies (the companies that made the original drug discovery). This requirement meant that very few generic medications entered the market because generic drug companies couldn't possibly recoup their R&D investments by selling low-cost generics.

The Hatch-Waxman legislation changed FDA regulations, allowing generic companies to rely on the originator company's efficacy data. In order to win FDA approval, the generic manufacturer now only has to demonstrate that its copycat product is both chemically and biologically identical to the brand. As a further incentive, the first company to produce a generic version is awarded 6 months of market exclusivity, meaning that no other generic companies are allowed to compete during that time. This is why it takes at least 6 months—and usually longer—for the price of a newly minted generic to fall.

Generic Drugs and Bioequivalence

The FDA requires generic drug makers to demonstrate that a generic is "biologically equivalent" to the brand-name drug that it will replace. In order to accomplish this, companies conduct studies in which 25–30 healthy volunteers take a single dose of both the brand and generic versions. Their blood is drawn sequentially, and the data are analyzed to obtain averages for Cmax (peak concentration level), AUC (area under the curve), half-life, and sometimes other variables (see Chapter 4 for an explanation of these quantities). The numbers obtained for the generic are then compared with those obtained for the brand-name drug, and this comparison forms the basis for an assessment of the bioequivalence of the two formulations.

FDA guidelines specify that the bioavailability of a generic must be, on average, between 80% and 125% of the original brand. Otherwise, the generic will not be approved. This may seem like a liberal amount of leeway, particularly for drugs that have a narrow therapeutic index, like antiseizure medications or antiarrhythmics. However, most generics achieve much better bioequivalence than this spread suggests. We know this because every few years the FDA reviews all the bioequivalence studies that generic companies have submitted. A review of such results from 1996 to 2007 found that the average difference between the AUC of generic and brand-name drugs was only 3.5% (Davit BM et al, *Ann Pharmacother* 2009;43(10):1583–1597). This implies that the bioavailability of, say, a 50 mg dose of generic sertraline is likely to deviate from 50 mg of Zoloft by no more than about 2 mg either way. A patient who is switched from 50 mg of Zoloft to 50 mg of generic sertraline may actually be absorbing between 48 mg and 52 mg QD—unlikely to be clinically significant in any but the most sensitive patients.

The FDA provides three rating categories for bioequivalence:

- AB: The generic has demonstrated bioequivalence to the brand in human studies
- AA: Human studies have not been done, but bioequivalence is likely
- B: The generic might not be bioequivalent

Almost all generic drugs have an AB rating. B-rated drugs, which represent about 4% of the market, are generally older drugs that have never been adequately tested. In many states, if you write "substitutions permitted" on a prescription, the pharmacist is mandated to fill it as a generic, but only if the generic is AB or AA rated.

"Authorized" and "Branded" Generics

As generic drugs have become more common and have taken more market share away from branded drugs, the originator drug companies have come up with ways to claw back some of that cash. Two prominent methods used by companies are to market authorized generics and branded generics.

An authorized generic is made by the same manufacturer of the original drug. An example is Pfizer's sertraline, which is produced on the same assembly line as the original Zoloft but stamped with the generic name "sertraline." Many patients who don't trust regular generics look for authorized generics and may ask you to prescribe them specifically. The only problem is that authorized generics are more expensive.

A branded generic is usually a pill made by a generic company, but instead of using the chemical name, the company comes up with a memorable brand name. For example, Methylin ER is a branded generic that is identical to methylphenidate sustained release. Other branded generics differ in trivial ways from the original medication, such as Aplenzin (bupropion) and Pexeva (paroxetine), which use different binding agents. The bottom line is that all this marketing doesn't change the fundamental pharmacology of the medication.

Generic Substitution: What Happens at the Pharmacy?

When you give a patient a prescription, do you write the brand or the generic name on the script? Many of us write the brand name because it's easier to remember and to write. But what happens when your patient brings the script to the pharmacy? The answer varies by state. A recent study in *JAMA Internal Medicine* reviewed all state laws and reported that only 19 states mandate pharmacies to substitute a generic for a branded medication if a generic is available (Sacks CA et al, *JAMA Intern Med* 2021;181(1):16–22). In the remaining 31 states, pharmacies "may" substitute. In seven states, pharmacies are required to get patient consent before a generic substitution. Requiring such consent lowers the generic substitution rate by about 25%—which translates to huge extra expenses borne by both our patients and insurance companies.

If you want to ensure that your patient receives the brand-name drug, you can do so by writing "dispense as written" on the script. But think twice before doing so. Your patients will likely end up spending more money, and research has shown that drug adherence and health outcomes are better on generic drugs because of the cost savings (Gagne JJ et al, *Ann Intern Med* 2014;161(6):400–407).

Generic Drugs in Psychiatry: A Review of the Research

Now that you know more about the generic drug industry, we'll review the research on whether specific generics are as efficacious as their branded brethren.

Most of the publications in this area are case reports and open-label studies, which are prone to the placebo effect—the exact kind of bias that makes patients and clinicians doubt the efficacy of generics to begin with.

The following study illustrates the problem. Researchers in New Zealand gathered 87 college students who suffered frequent headaches and randomized them to ibuprofen or placebo. The treatments were delivered in two phases. In the first, both the placebo and the ibuprofen were stamped "generic ibuprofen." With that stamp, the active treatment worked much better than the placebo. Next, researchers revved up the power of suggestion by labeling both the placebo and the real ibuprofen with a brand name. The power of suggestion overwhelmed the true medication effect; the "branded" placebo worked just as well as the real, branded ibuprofen. This type of study has been repeated in many variations, sometimes finding that medications are better tolerated when stamped with a brand name (Faasse K et al, *Health Psychol* 2016;35(2):187–190).

TABLE 16-1. Generic Stumbles Over the Years

Clozapine	There were reports of increased relapses when patients switched from brand to generic clozapine in 2001, particularly with the Zenith generic (later bought by Teva). A more recent analysis concluded this problem is very rare and best managed by measuring the serum levels.
Concerta	Two generic versions tended to dump too much of the dose in the morning and run out of therapeutic efficacy by afternoon (they are no longer considered generic equivalents of Concerta).
Bupropion and venlafaxine	Some of the generic extended-release versions of these antidepressants—venlafaxine XR and Budeprion XL—had a tendency to dump the entire dose shortly after taking it, resulting in side effects in the morning and withdrawal problems in the afternoon. Both were made by Teva. The problematic Budeprion XL has since been withdrawn from the market.
Anticonvulsants	Anticonvulsants have a narrower therapeutic window in epilepsy than bipolar disorder. Hence, there are reports of increased seizures after switching to generic lamotrigine, carbamazepine, and valproate, but this has not clearly translated to problems in bipolar disorder.
Levothyroxine	A manufacturing problem led to a generic form of Synthroid that was not bioequivalent to the brand. This was corrected, as demonstrated in a 1997 study.

In order to truly test generics, we'd need to randomly assign patients to continuing on the brand vs switching, and we'd need to make sure that both the doctors and the patients are unaware of which patients are getting which treatment (a so-called randomized double-blind study). In this brief review, we'll focus on a few medications that have been well researched or have been the subject of particular scrutiny.

Clozapine and the Antipsychotics

Soon after generic clozapine was approved in 1999, several case reports appeared describing reemergence of psychotic symptoms after switching from Clozaril to clozapine. Soon, both Novartis (the manufacturer of Clozaril) and generic manufacturers commissioned large studies that compared Clozaril with generic clozapine. The results of these studies depended on the source of funding. There was a neat split between the studies funded by Novartis, which reported that patients who were switched to generic clozapine did poorly (Kluznik JC et al, *J Clin Psychiatry* 2001;62[Suppl 5]:14–17; Mofsen R and Balter J, *Clin Ther* 2001;23(10):1720–1731), and the studies funded by generic companies, which reported that the generic was well tolerated (Makela EH et al, *Ann Pharmacother* 2003;37(3):350–353; Stoner SC et al, *Pharmacotherapy* 2003;23(6):806–810). The Novartis-funded studies caused a significant ruckus, and the FDA responded by requesting the generic makers to repeat their bioequivalence research, which they did, apparently to the FDA's satisfaction.

Two larger studies have looked at the question without any industry funding—brand company or generic. Both appear to exonerate generic clozapine. These were retrospective studies that followed close to 400 patients for 3–6 months after the Clozaril-to-clozapine switch. In both reports, the patients either improved clinically or showed no change after the switch (Paton C, *Br J Psychiatry* 2006;189:184–185; Alessi-Severini S et al, *J Clin Psychiatry* 2006;67(7):1047–1054).

Outside of clozapine, studies from New Zealand and Italy tracked health care utilization before and after large numbers of patients were switched from branded to generic olanzapine and risperidone. Switching to generic did not change use of outpatient or inpatient services (Blier P et al, *Int J Psychiatry Clin Pract* 2019;23(1):2–13).

The bottom line is that large-scale studies conducted by investigators without commercial conflicts of interest indicate that generic clozapine is as safe and effective as brand-name Clozaril.

Antidepressants

A few studies have used large national databases to look at whether patients are more likely to require hospital admission after switching to generic antidepressants. The results have been mixed and are difficult to interpret because of the lack of randomization. In such studies, you also can't control for the possibility that the patients who remained on brand-name drugs may have also received higher-quality treatment in other ways. The most careful study concluded that any difference in hospitalization rates was reflective of perception bias against generics rather than a difference in the biological actions of formulations (Desai RJ et al, *PLoS Med* 2019;16(3):e1002763).

Turning to individual antidepressants, a New Zealand study compared 12,407 patients who stayed on brand-name Effexor XR to 1,624 who switched to generic venlafaxine XR between 2011 and 2013. There was no difference in any measure of health care utilization between the two groups (Lessing C et al, *Value Health* 2015;18(5):646–654).

There is one report from 2007 of worsened panic, mood, and suicidality in 20 out of 172 patients (12%) with anxiety disorders who switched from branded Celexa to generic citalopram. The patients were not aware of the switch, and they improved with return to the brand, with some needing a dose increase (Van Ameringen M et al, *J Psychopharmacol* 2007;21(5):472–476).

More serious problems occurred with a certain generic Wellbutrin. In the 2006, Teva released Budeprion XL, the first generic version of Wellbutrin XL. As required, they submitted their bioequivalence studies to the FDA, but with a catch. They only turned in documents for the 150 mg dose, and the FDA assumed that the 300 mg was also comparable. It was not. Patients started lobbying the FDA with complaints of dizziness, depression, and suicidality after making the switch. The FDA reassured them that the product was sound, until a public radio host—Joe Graedon of *The People's Pharmacy*—got involved and forced the agency to retest the capsules. When they did, they found the 300 mg was dose dumping, releasing most of its contents early in the day, which was causing patients to have morning toxicity and afternoon withdrawal. Budeprion XL 300 mg was pulled from the market in 2012, but the 150 mg tablet lives on.

The bottom line is that extended-release formulations are harder for generic companies to copy. The companies that develop these complex formulations are not required to reveal their manufacturing secrets, so generic companies have to reverse-engineer the pill.

Anticonvulsants

As opposed to antidepressants and anxiolytics, there is a fair amount of literature on brand vs generic anticonvulsants, but most of this involves epilepsy. A meta-analysis of such studies published in 2010 found no differences in clinical outcomes between the two formulations (Kesselheim AS et al, *Drugs* 2010;70(5):605–621). As is often the case in this literature, case reports find that switching to generics leads to problems, but subsequent larger studies report equivalence. For example, some case reports had indicated complications or breakthrough seizures after patients were switched from Tegretol to generic carbamazepine, but two rigorous double-blind comparisons showed no differences in bioavailability or clinical efficacy (Oles KS et al, *Neurology* 1992;42(6):1147–1153; Silpakit O et al, *Ann Pharmacother* 1997;31(5):548–552).

Psychostimulants

In 2016 the FDA determined that two generic versions of Concerta (manufactured by Mallinckrodt and UCB/Kremers Urban) were not as effective as the branded product and downgraded their approval from the bioequivalent "AB" to the non-equivalent "BX," which means pharmacies are discouraged from automatically substituting these for the branded version. The decision makes sense, as these non-equivalent versions do not utilize the same OROS delivery system as Concerta and were less effective than Concerta in a small, independently founded clinical trial (Lally MD et al, *Clin Pediatr (Phila)* 2016;55(13):1197–1201).

Currently there are several generic versions of Concerta that are still considered equivalent to the original, including an authorized generic from Janssen and a regular generic from Mylan. You don't have to specify "brand name only" for Concerta because pharmacies cannot automatically switch to a substandard BX generic. As an added precaution you can write "OROS delivery system only" on the script.

Benzodiazepines

In terms of research on generic benzodiazepines, there is a published report challenging the anecdotal impression that generic clonazepam is less effective than branded Klonopin. This report is contained in a letter from a psychiatrist concerning two of his private-practice patients. In both patients, the generic version actually was *more* anxiolytic and sedating than the brand-name version, exactly opposite to common opinion (Rapaport MH, *J Clin Psychopharmacol* 1997;17(5):424).

Thyroid Medication

Psychiatrists sometimes prescribe thyroid medications to treat hypothyroidism, as can happen on lithium, or as an augmentation strategy in unipolar or bipolar depression. But there's a lot of controversy about which type of thyroid supplement to use and whether to stick with the brand or generic.

The thyroid gland produces two thyroid hormones: thyroxine (T4) and triiodothyronine (T3). Each of these is available on pharmacy shelves as levothyroxine (Synthroid, T4) and liothyronine (Cytomel, T3), two synthetically manufactured analogues of the original hormones. A third version is also available—dessicated thyroid—which contains a mix of T4 and T3 extracted from pig glands and is sold under various brands, including Armour Thyroid and Nature-Throid.

Patients who prefer natural treatments often opt for dessicated thyroid, but endocrinologists generally discourage this route because pigs have 3 times more T3 than humans. T3 is the more potent of the two thyroid hormones, and excessive T3 from dessicated products has been known to cause symptoms of hyperthyroidism like anxiety, insomnia, and tachycardia (McAninch EA and Bianco AC, *Front Endocrinol (Lausanne)* 2019;10:446). Instead, endocrinologists recommend levothyroxine as the first-line treatment for hypothyroidism. Levothyroxine is converted in the liver into triiodothyronine (T3) at a rate that generally resembles the normal ratio of T4:T3, so it is usually not necessary to supplement with both (Garber JR et al, *Thyroid* 2012;22(12):1200–1235).

But the controversy does not end there. Levothyroxine has long been mired in debate over the bioequivalence between the generic and the brand (Synthroid). The problem began in 1980 when a paper in *JAMA* exposed the discrepancy between the two formulations. Several subsequent papers suggested the problem had been corrected, but the issue was revived in the 1990s when the FDA recalled several levothyroxine products because their strength did not match their labeling (Dong BJ et al, *JAMA* 1997;277(15):1205–1213). The problem was so widespread that the FDA decided to hit the reset button in 1997, requiring all manufacturers of levothyroxine to resubmit their products for approval.

We'd like to report that the controversy ended there, but product recalls and problematic studies of brand vs generic levothyroxine continue. As this book was going to press, a 16-year study of 19,850 patients who either stayed on the brand or switched to generic appeared. Those who stayed on Synthroid were more likely to have stable TSH levels and less likely to develop clinical consequences of hypothyroidism like depression, obesity, hypertension, and renal disease (Hennessey JV et al, *Adv Ther* 2021;38(1):337–349).

Part of the problem is that levothyroxine is a delicate compound that tends to degrade when exposed to excess light, heat, or moisture. Even if the medication is intact, it may not get all the way into your patient's system because foods rich in fiber or calcium interfere with its absorption.

While endocrinologists prefer levothyroxine, psychiatric experts are split on whether levothyroxine (T4) or liothyronine (T3) should be used in depression. Liothyronine has more potent effects in the CNS and is supported by a taller stack of clinical studies. Those who prefer levothyroxine argue that it is more in line with the normal balance of the two hormones. We don't claim to have the final answer on these issues, but here is some basic guidance:

1. If you are treating hypothyroidism, start with levothyroxine—either generic or brand—and refer to an endocrinologist if the thyroid panel does not stabilize.

2. If your patient has normal thyroid function and you are adding a thyroid supplement to treat depression, either levothyroxine or liothyronine could work, but the steps are complex and you should familiarize yourself with them first. Tammas Kelly's 2018 book *The Art and Science of Thyroid Supplementation for the Treatment of Bipolar Depression* is a good start.

Looking back at all the classes of generic psychiatric medications we've just reviewed, the published literature is not robust enough to draw any definitive conclusions. Readers have likely developed their own clinical feelings for which generics are more or less likely to result in patient phone calls, and this may be the best "information" we have at this point.

Patent Extenders: A Growth Industry

Because the pipeline for novel psychotropic medications has been relatively dry, many drug companies resort to evergreening their medications by reformulating them into patentable variations on the original product.

Typical evergreening techniques include:

1. Introducing an extended-release medication
2. Introducing a purified stereoisomer of a racemic medication—eg, esketamine (Spravato) is the S-isomer of ketamine
3. Introducing the active metabolite of a medication—eg, desvenlafaxine is a metabolite of venlafaxine and paliperidone is a metabolite of risperidone
4. Introducing a new indication for an old medication—eg, Silenor is doxepin approved in a lower dosage for insomnia

In conjunction with creating a patent extender, there are certain marketing techniques commonly used by companies to "migrate" prescriptions from the old version of a drug to the new version:

1. The company introduces the new formulation at least one year *before* the old formulation goes generic and uses this time to migrate clinicians to the brand-name drug
2. Drug reps stop sampling the old version before it becomes generic to discourage its use
3. All promotions of the old version cease, and ads and industry-funded continuing medical education programs focus entirely on the advantages of the "novel" formulation
4. The drug company often increases the price of the soon-to-go-generic version in order to make the higher price of the new version less of a shock to insurance companies

That methodology may seem manipulative at best, but does it mean the new product is not worth prescribing? We've summed up the pros and cons

TABLE 16-2. Recent Patent Extenders in Psychiatry

Original Drug	New Drug	Putative Advantages	The Catch
Asenapine (Saphris)	Secuado (skin patch)	Improved adherence	No data to support this claim
Aripiprazole (Abilify)	Abilify MyCite	Tracks adherence with a microchip	Complex instructions that require patients to wear a signal-transducing patch that is replaced weekly and paired to their smartphone; the claims of improved adherence are unproven
Aripiprazole (Abilify)	Brexpiprazole (Rexulti, a structural analogue of aripiprazole)	Lower D_2 affinity, lower rates of akathisia and sedation	Head-to-head comparisons are lacking
Quetiapine (Seroquel)	Quetiapine XR (Seroquel XR)	Less sedation and orthostasis, once-a-day dosing	The original can usually be dosed all at night, and when dosed this way it is no more sedating than XR
Risperidone (Risperdal)	Invega (paliperidone, an active metabolite of risperidone)	Fewer drug interactions, no need for titration	None
Lamotrigine (Lamictal)	Lamictal XR (lamotrigine XR)	Steady serum levels may prevent breakthrough seizures	This benefit is not relevant in psychiatry
Duloxetine (Cymbalta)	Cymbalta sprinkles	Easier to swallow	None
Venlafaxine (Effexor)	Pristiq (desvenlafaxine, an active metabolite of venlafaxine)	Dose titration not necessary, fewer withdrawal problems, fewer drug interactions	None
Dextroamphetamine	Vyvanse (lisdexamfetamine, a metabolic precursor of dextroamphetamine)	Lower risk of abuse	None; Vyvanse is due to go generic in 2023
Methylphenidate	Jornay PM	This delayed-release stimulant is dosed before bedtime so it kicks in as soon as the patient wakes up	Dubious relevance

(table continues)

of recent patent extenders as best we can in Table 16-2. A few, like brexpiprazole (Rexulti), desvenlafaxine (Pristiq), and lisdexamfetamine (Vyvanse) appear to offer real advantages, though head-to-head comparisons with the original are usually lacking. For most of the others, we are hard pressed to find a rationale that justifies their cost.

TABLE 16-2. Recent Patent Extenders in Psychiatry *(continued)*

Original Drug	New Drug	Putative Advantages	The Catch
Methylphenidate and amphetamine	Adhansia XR (methylphenidate) and Mydayis (amphetamine)	16-hour durations	Similar effects are achieved by adding an instant-release stimulant at the end of the day to a generic MR with a 12-hour duration
Doxepin	Silenor	Only the branded form is available in dosages appropriate for insomnia (3–6 mg)	Generic liquid doxepin does the job (1/8 teaspoon of 10 mg/mL doxepin = 6 mg)
Bupropion/ naltrexone	Contrave (bupropion/ naltrexone combination for weight loss)	This branded combo pill packs both medications in an extended-release capsule at doses that are difficult to replicate (8–32 mg naltrexone + 90–360 mg bupropion)	The two have been successfully used as separate pills in a few studies (naltrexone instant release 50 mg + bupropion XL 300 mg)[1]

[1] Grilo CM et al, *Clin Ther* 2021;43(1):112–122.e1

CHAPTER 17

Pharmacogenetic Testing

WHETHER YOU BELIEVE THAT PHARMACOGENETIC testing is useful or not, you'll need to know how to interpret these brave new tests. These days, patients are showing up for their first consultation with results in hand. In this chapter, we'll review the concepts driving these tests as well as the research on whether, at the end of the day, they are actually useful.

Pharmacokinetic Genes, Pharmacodynamic Genes, and Their Combinations

Genetic tests look at two types of genes:

1. *Pharmacokinetic genes* alter the levels of drugs, either through metabolic enzymes in the liver or as the drugs pass through the blood-brain barrier.
2. *Pharmacodynamic genes* shape the body's response to medications. These include genes for neurotransmitter receptors and genes that predict side effects.

Pharmacokinetic Genes: The CYP450 System

First, let's review our molecular biology. Enzymes are proteins, which are made up of amino acids. Amino acids, in turn, are put together according to the sequences of nucleotide base pairs in our DNA. A *gene* refers to a specific sequence of nucleotide base pairs leading to the formation of a specific compound.

Each of the cytochrome P450 (CYP450) enzymes is built by a particular gene. Individuals vary in their genetic makeup, and this variability doesn't end with obvious characteristics like eye color and height. In fact, there is inter-individual variability, or *polymorphism*, in the genes coding for CYP450 enzymes.

Genes lie on chromosomes, and chromosomes come in pairs: one from the mother and one from the father. This means that each gene comes in two copies, or *alleles*, and it is the variations in these alleles that make us—and our CYP450 enzymes—unique. As an example, the gene coding for the CYP450 2D6 enzyme is carried on our 22nd chromosome. Most people have two normal alleles (ie, copies) of the 2D6 gene: one on each of their two #22 chromosomes. This allows each copy to produce the enzyme, ensuring that we have a good supply and are able to transform substrates of 2D6 at the expected rate. Based on the CYP450 polymorphisms, individuals are categorized in different ways with respect to specific enzymes:

- *Extensive metabolizers*, otherwise known as "normal" metabolizers, have normally active CYP450 genes on both chromosomes, meaning their serum drug levels rise to average, expected levels.
- *Intermediate metabolizers* have only one working copy of a CYP450 gene or two copies that are only partially working, causing them to metabolize drugs a little slower than normal. However, there is controversy about whether we should really be concerned about this category, which encompasses about 40% of Caucasians and has similar rates in most other populations. Although dosage adjustments may not be necessary in intermediate metabolizers, they are more vulnerable to drug interactions at those enzymes. Even a weak drug interaction could turn an intermediate metabolizer into the next category: poor metabolizer.
- *Poor metabolizers* carry inactive or partially active CYP450 genes, and therefore metabolize drugs significantly slower than extensive metabolizers. This may result in more side effects because the serum drug levels are higher. The effect is similar to taking a drug that is a potent inhibitor at that enzyme. About 7%–10% of most populations are poor metabolizers, but for Asians the rates are much higher (20%–40%).
- *Ultrarapid metabolizers* have extra copies of certain genes and therefore metabolize drugs more quickly than extensive metabolizers, sometimes requiring unusually high doses of medications to achieve a therapeutic level. The effect is similar to taking a medication that is a potent inducer at the enzyme.

There are a number of CYP450 enzymes—for example, 1A2, 2D6, 2C19, and 3A4. A person can be a poor metabolizer at one enzyme, but an extensive metabolizer at another.

Is Metabolizer Status Clinically Relevant?

The short answer is yes, but only for certain medications. The FDA keeps an updated list of medications where the research is reliable enough to support pharmacogenetic-guided dosing. As with many things in psychiatry, older drugs are at a disadvantage on this list because they lack well-heeled backers to support their research. We've summarized the FDA list in Table 17-1, and you can check for updates at www. fda.gov/medical-devices/precision-medicine/table-pharmacogenetic-associations.

Poor metabolizers generally require lower dosages to achieve a therapeutic level and may have significant side effects in the normal dose range. In practice, that may show up as tremor, fatigue, or akathisia, but the side effect that concerns the FDA most is QTc prolongation. Although rare, this risk is potentially fatal, and the life-threatening arrhythmias it can cause are more likely to occur at higher serum levels. For that reason, the FDA requires CYP testing at high doses of pimozide and recommends it for thioridazine, citalopram, and the tardive dyskinesia medications deutetrabenazine and valbenazine. Those drugs have dosing and/or frequency restrictions for poor metabolizers, and thioridazine is contraindicated in poor metabolizers (see Table 17-1, and yes—the FDA is a little inconsistent in their directions, which require us to take specific actions in the presence of a known test result, but only require us to order that test with pimozide).

If you do prescribe a medication in Table 17-1 to a poor metabolizer, the directions are similar to what you would do if they were taking a strong inhibitor. Start at half the usual dose of the medication and raise it twice as slowly as you normally would. Lower the target dose by 30%–70%. For rapid metabolizers, the risk is different—it's efficacy rather than tolerability we worry about here. So while you could titrate the dose faster, you might just stick with a normal titration if side effects are a significant concern. But you would aim for a higher target dose, about 135%–180% higher (see Table 17-2).

Keep the medications in Table 17-1 in mind when a patient calls with unusually severe side effects. If they've recently started a drug in the table, they may be a poor metabolizer and testing is warranted. A study of atomoxetine (Eugene AR, *PeerJ* 2020;8:e8748) illustrates the point. This ADHD medication causes sedation in about 1 in 20 patients, but it ranked near the top of medications with an antidepressant structure that triggered reports of sedation to the FDA's surveillance system. How did a rare side

TABLE 17-1. Pharmacogenetic Recommendations From the FDA

	Medication	Gene	Risk	Action
Testing Required	Carbamazepine (and possibly oxcarbazepine)	HLA-B*1502	Stevens-Johnson syndrome (SJS)	In patients of Asian descent, test is required before starting carbamazepine and recommended before oxcarbazepine; a positive result in this population means they are 80 times more likely to develop SJS on carbamazepine and 30 times more likely on oxcarbazepine
	Pimozide	2D6	Arrhythmias	Test is required before dosing pimozide above 4 mg/day (or 0.05 mg/kg/day in children) because of risk of arrhythmias; in poor metabolizers, wait 14 days between dose adjustments
Testing Recommended	Thioridazine	2D6	Arrhythmias	Contraindicated in poor metabolizers
	Citalopram	2C19	Arrhythmias	Max dose of 20 mg/day in poor metabolizers
	Deutetrabenazine (Austedo)	2D6	Arrhythmias	Max dose 18 mg BID in poor metabolizers (BID dosing is required in this population)
	Valbenazine (Ingrezza)	2D6	Arrhythmias	Lower the dose by 50% and divide it twice a day in poor metabolizers
Adjust the Dose if Testing Results Are Known	Atomoxetine, clozapine, perphenazine, venlafaxine, vortioxetine (Trintellix), and various tricyclics (amitriptyline, clomipramine, desipramine, doxepin, imipramine, nortriptyline, protriptyline, trimipramine)	2D6	Various	Lower the dose by 50% in poor metabolizers; for clozapine and tricyclics, adjust based on serum levels; for venlafaxine, keep in mind that the active metabolite (desvenlafaxine) will be low in poor metabolizers and high in rapid metabolizers
	Aripiprazole, brexpiprazole (Rexulti), iloperidone	2D6, 3A4	Various	Lower the dose by 50% in poor metabolizers at either enzyme, or by 75% if both enzymes are poor
	Flibanserin (Addyi)	3A4	Syncope	Lower the dose in poor metabolizers
	Lumateperone (Caplyta)	3A4	Various	Lower the dose in poor metabolizers

Sources: www.cpicpgx.org/genes-drugs; www.fda.gov/drugs/science-and-research-drugs/table-pharmacogenomic-biomarkers-drug-labeling

TABLE 17-2. Dosing Adjustments for Pharmacokinetic Genes

Result	What It Means	Dosing Adjustment
Extensive (normal) metabolizer	Metabolic clearance is unchanged	Nothing different
Poor (slow) metabolizer	Metabolic clearance is severely slowed, raising the levels of drugs that go through the pathway	Lower the dose by 30%–70%
Intermediate metabolizer	Metabolic clearance is moderately slowed, which may or may not raise the levels of drugs that go through the pathway	Watch carefully, as dose reductions may or may not be in order; the patient will be more prone to drug interactions if they take medications that further inhibit the enzyme
Ultrarapid metabolizer	Metabolic clearance is accelerated, lowering the levels of drugs that go through the pathway	Raise the dose by 135%–180%

effect make it to the top of the list? Atomoxetine levels peak 10-fold higher in poor CYP2D6 metabolizers, so with this drug, when it rains, it pours.

Genes for Drug Allergies

Among the genes recommended by the FDA, one of them is not like the others: HLA-B*1502. This gene has no effect on drug metabolism (ie, pharmacokinetics), but it does predict whether certain drugs will cause a serious rash (a pharmacodynamic effect).

Patients who are positive for HLA-B*1502 are 80 times more likely to develop Stevens-Johnson syndrome (SJS) on carbamazepine, 30 times more likely to develop it on oxcarbazepine, and twice as likely with lamotrigine. There are also reports of increased risk of SJS with use of phenytoin. HLA-B*1502 is virtually absent in non-Asian patients, so the FDA only requires the test before prescribing carbamazepine to patients of Asian descent. For oxcarbazepine, the test is recommended (not required) in Asian patients, and for lamotrigine the FDA does not even mention the test, as a positive result would only change the odds of a severe rash from 1 in 3,000 to 2 in 3,000.

Specific groups with elevated rates (10%–15%) of HLA-B*1502 include Hong Kong, Thailand, Malaysia, China, Taiwan, and the Philippines; rates are lower (2%–4%) in South Asia, India, and North China, and lower still (< 1%) in Japan and Korea.

There is another genetic test that predicts liver failure on valproic acid, but this gene (polymerase gamma or POLG) is only present in patients with hereditary neurometabolic syndromes like Alpers-Huttenlocher syndrome. The FDA requires testing for POLG before prescribing valproic acid in those patients.

From Genetic Tests to Pharmacogenomic Algorithms

So far we've made a case for testing single genes in very specific situations, but you don't need to order a pharmacogenetic panel to check them. A simple blood test at most clinical laboratories will suffice. These tests don't inspire any controversy, but when we turn to commercial pharmacogenetic panels, things get more heated.

Commercial pharmacogenetic panels offer something quite distinct from the pat-and-dry recommendations above. These tests use proprietary algorithms that sort through dozens of genes to guide the selection of drugs for depression, schizophrenia, and ADHD. Many of them have been subject to clinical trials, and for the most part, the results don't look very good.

In the early studies, these genetic panels appeared effective. Patients got better when their antidepressants were chosen based on the genetic results, much better than treatment as usual. But those studies were unblinded, which leaves open the possibility that the high-tech aura of the test was simply amplifying the placebo effect. Results of blinded studies have been less impressive, but clever proponents often present the data in misleading ways, so it's worth reviewing them.

Most of these studies started with patients who had not responded to their first antidepressant. That kind of "enriched sample" should favor the test, as these patients are more likely to have genetic variations that interfered with their treatment. Next, they randomized those patients to receive a second antidepressant that was either guided or unguided by the pharmacogenomic algorithm. Although the patients were not aware of whether their genetic tests were used to guide their treatment, their doctors were, and it's possible that those doctors prescribed the gene-guided medications with a touch more enthusiasm.

Several large trials like this have been conducted, and all but one has had equivocal results. By "equivocal," we mean the benefits of the test were so small that it took a lot of statistical maneuvering to brush them up. The sole positive one was the Amplis test from CNSDose, which takes a different approach from the other panels. Amplis looks at genes for the p-glycoprotein transporter, which transports some medications across the blood-brain barrier. We'll get to that in a minute.

Among the panels with negative results are AssureRx's GeneSight, Genomind's Genecept, AltheaDx's NeuroIDgenetix, and Genpharm's Neuropharmagen. These tests made no difference on the primary outcome—depression—in trials involving thousands of patients. But they did produce some positive results on secondary measures and post-hoc analyses where the sample was divided up in various ways (aka "data fishing"). That kind of analysis is meant to inform future studies, not clinical practice, because the findings may have been arrived at by chance. Chance, and its statistical cousin probability, are supposed to keep medical research in check, but they haven't kept these secondary findings from glossing the covers of the pharmacogenetic promotional brochures.

Even if these secondary outcomes are valid, they are not very impressive. With GeneSight's secondary measures, you'd need to test 19 patients to bring 1 to remission. If their sample was limited to the minority of patients who actually had genetic variations that informed the medication choice, those figures improve slightly: You'd need to test 13 patients to bring 1 to remission.

One reason behind the disappointing performance of these panels may have to do with their reliance on pharmacodynamic genes. Those genes are supposed to tell us how the brain responds to medications, but there is scant evidence that any of them actually do. In the sidebar, we've detailed the most famous of these pharmacodynamic genes: the short arm of the serotonin receptor.

Another problem may lie in the accuracy of the test results. A study where samples were sent to different direct-to-consumer laboratories showed inconsistency between the companies in the specific genotypes as well as in the metabolic phenotypes—meaning whether they thought a given patient was a poor, intermediate, or rapid metabolizer. And the medications that

The Serotonin Transporter Gene

While pharmacokinetic genes tell us about dosing, pharmacodynamic genes tell us how medications might act once they get into the brain. It's a tantalizing idea, but one that has proven unreliable in clinical trials. In the brain, a single gene can act in opposite directions depending on the environment it was raised in and the other genes it is paired with.

The serotonin reuptake transporter (aka "SERT" or "5-HTT") gene is the best studied in the pharmacodynamic lot. The gene that codes for SERT is SLC6A4, and that's the term you'll probably see on a genetic panel. SLC6A4 comes in two sizes, or alleles: short (S) and long (L). People with two S alleles have fewer serotonin transporters. Why does this matter? Well, it's from this receptor that selective serotonin reuptake inhibitors (SSRIs) get their name. SERT is where the SSRIs do their work, blocking serotonin reuptake.

According to pharmacogenetic tests, people with the short (S/S) allele are less likely to respond to SSRIs and more likely to have side effects on them. The idea makes sense, because they have fewer receptors to act on. However, most meta-analyses have failed to support it (Porcelli S et al, *Eur Neuropsychopharmacol* 2012;22(4):239–258). At best, it seems to hold up only in Caucasians, particularly those who are older or male. This makes some biological sense. Estrogen increases SERT expression, so we might expect the S/S allele to have a more marked effect on SERT in men and post-menopausal women.

SERT also made headlines in 2003 after a study found that people with the S/S allele were more likely to get depressed under stress (Caspi A et al, *Science* 2003;301(5631):386–369). That finding has since bounced back and forth with positive and negative results in over 50 studies, and it has not held up in most meta-analyses.

There are other pharmacodynamic genes you may encounter in practice, like BDNF, HTR2, COMT, and MTHFR. The rationale behind their use is based more on theory than clinical evidence. Some had early positive results, but fell prey to a common trend—the more a gene is studied, the less those results tend to hold up.

they recommended or cautioned against were very different (Bousman CA et al, *Pharmacogenet Genomics* 2017;27(11):387–393). The FDA has gone so far as to issue cease-and-desist letters to some of these companies. While genotyping panels may become helpful in the future, the lack of standardization alone is enough reason to avoid them. Instead, we recommend ordering specific genes from reliable laboratories when indicated.

CNSDose: Pharmacokinetics at the Blood-Brain Barrier

The only genetic panel with a positive study is one that focuses on pharmacokinetics rather than pharmacodynamics: CNSDose's Amplis. It includes the FDA's favorite CYP genes (2D6 and 2C19), as well as UGT1A1, which metabolizes desvenlafaxine. But what really sets it apart are the genes for the p-glycoprotein transporter: ABCB1 and ABCC1.

Just as the CYP enzymes kick some medications out of the body, p-glycoprotein kicks some of them out of the brain. If the patient has genetic variations that upregulate p-glycoprotein's activity, they will need higher doses of those medications to get them past this bouncer and into the CNS. The problem is that you need to bring the serum level very high to get the CNS level to normal, which means more physical side effects. A better solution is to switch to a medication that isn't affected by p-glycoprotein.

The study that put CNSDose on the map was a randomized controlled trial of 148 patients with depression. Half had gene-guided treatment, and the other half did not. Only the treating physician, not the patients or the raters, knew who was in which group. After 12 weeks, remission rates were much higher in the gene-guided cohort. How high? You'd need to test 3 patients to bring 1 to remission. Those are pretty good odds, but they need replication (Singh AB, *Clin Psychopharmacol Neurosci* 2015;13(2):150–156).

Even if you don't run this panel, it's good to know which antidepressants don't depend on p-glycoprotein as these may be worth trying in treatment-resistant cases. They include bupropion, duloxetine, fluoxetine, and mirtazapine. Medications that do depend on this transporter are listed in Table 17-3.

Like the CYP system, p-glycoprotein is also subject to drug interactions, although the research here is not as well developed as it is for CYP450. P-glycoprotein inhibitors prevent the transporter from pumping its substrate drugs out of the brain, leading to more CNS effects, while inducers will do the opposite, rendering p-glycoprotein substrates ineffective. Strong inducers include carbamazepine, phenytoin, rifampin, and St. John's wort. Strong inhibitors include amiodarone, clarithromycin, erythromycin, itraconazole, quinidine, ritonavir, and verapamil.

TABLE 17-3. Medications Impacted by P-Glycoprotein

	P-Glycoprotein Substrates
SSRI	Citalopram, escitalopram, fluvoxamine, paroxetine, sertraline
SNRI	Desvenlafaxine, reboxetine, venlafaxine
TCA	Doxepin, amitriptyline, imipramine, nortriptyline, trimipramine
Antipsychotics	Risperidone, paliperidone

Can Genetic Testing Do More Harm Than Good?

Genetic testing may be helpful in some cases, such as in patients with unexplained poor responses or with unusually high vulnerability to side effects. But can ordering such tests paradoxically make outcomes worse? There are various scenarios in which it might:

- **Hasty medication switches.** Both GeneSight and Genecept produce reports in which they place recommended drugs in a green column labeled "use as directed" and others in a red or orange column labeled "use with caution." The company's marketing literature paints a rosy picture of treatment-resistant patients who have finally found the right medication as a result of these recommendations. But more skeptical press coverage has reported on patients who have done poorly, such as a man who was switched from venlafaxine to levomilnacipran and soon became acutely suicidal and was admitted to a hospital (www. tinyurl.com/hxkoyh8). We've seen fluoxetine show up in the red in children with the short arm of the SERT gene, but the bulk of the clinical evidence suggests that fluoxetine is the antidepressant most likely to work in this age group.
- **Inappropriate medication avoidance.** Practitioners might avoid potentially helpful medications based on the results of unproven tests. For example, certain SERT alleles will place all SSRIs in the "avoid"

box, but those same alleles indicate a favorable response to SSRIs in Asian patients.

- **Unwarranted patient skepticism.** Patients who read their reports will likely be skeptical of any drug in the discouraged category, making it difficult for you to prescribe them that drug in the future.

- **Premature assumptions that "normal" metabolizers are in the clear.** If a patient's results show that they are a normal metabolizer (eg, extensive or intermediate), you may be inclined to believe that you can dose the patient more aggressively without side effects. But in real-world patients, even normal metabolizers can end up with high serum levels. For example, in one study a large group of patients who took venlafaxine were genotyped, and 4% of them were poor metabolizers at CYP2D6. Researchers then focused on the 96% of patients who were not poor metabolizers, and surprisingly 27% of them had high ratios of venlafaxine to its metabolite—the pattern you'd expect in poor metabolizers. In some cases, patients were taking other drugs that decreased venlafaxine metabolism, but in other cases there was no clear explanation. The authors point out that genetic testing can be misleading, and that a person's actual metabolic abilities will vary based on nongenetic factors (Preskhorn SH et al, *J Clin Psychiatry* 2013;74(6):614–621).

VERDICTS

1. Avoid GeneSight, Genecept, and most other commercial panels. They aren't proven, and they might lead you to make inappropriate or potentially harmful prescribing decisions.

2. Keep your eye on CNSDose. If its initial spectacular results can be replicated, the test may be worth trying.

3. If you are the type of practitioner who likes to follow every FDA recommendation to the T, you might consider selectively ordering genotyping for specific enzymes, depending on the drug you are prescribing. But slow dose titration will accomplish the same purpose more cheaply.

4. If you are considering prescribing carbamazepine or oxcarbazepine to a person of Asian descent, you should test for the HLA-B*1502 allele. Avoid those medications if the results are positive, as the risk of Stevens-Johnson syndrome is just too high.

CHAPTER 18

Prescribing for the Elderly and the Young

AS IF LIFE WEREN'T COMPLICATED enough for a hard-working psychopharmacologist these days, we have to add yet another factor to our decision-making—the fact that various aspects of drug metabolism vary with age.

We'll start at the end of the story, with the elderly, because we know so much more about drug metabolism in this age group. The elderly receive much more medical treatment than the young, which has led to a larger body of research on drug disposition in elderly patients. Elderly patients are generally taking multiple medications, with more complex drug-drug interactions. There is often a prescribing cascade, where patients are given medications for symptoms that are side effects of other medications. Psychopharmacologic treatment of children, relatively speaking, is in its infancy.

Drug Metabolism in the Elderly

Absorption

About 1 in 20 elderly patients have significant problems with drug absorption. One reason is that the number of intestinal absorptive cells in the GI system decrease with age, but the effect is not very predictable. Those who are affected may come to your attention because they don't seem to be responding to adequate doses of medication. You can check a serum level to see if a decent amount of the medication is getting into the bloodstream, which is useful to know even if the therapeutic range of the drug is not well defined.

Orally disintegrating tablets (ODTs) may help in these cases, and ODTs are also useful for another problem that is common in the elderly:

swallowing. The elderly are more likely to suffer from dysphagia, particularly if they have had a stroke, Parkinson's disease, or poorly fitting dentures. Ask your elderly patients if they have swallowing difficulties, and if they do, ask if they would prefer an ODT formulation.

Distribution

Recall from Chapter 3 that the elderly tend to have a higher proportion of adipose tissue (due to age-related decline in muscle mass), and this increases the volume of distribution. Most medications are lipophilic, so they are drawn into this fatty tissue and away from the bloodstream, rendering them less effective.

Thus with initial doses of drugs, plasma levels may actually be *lower* in the elderly than in younger patients. The catch, however, is that because the drug is stored in fat, it stays around longer, meaning that its effective half-life is longer. Combine this with the fact that the rate of clearance of drugs is often lower in the elderly (due to factors such as decreased blood flow to the liver and decreased glomerular filtration rate), and you can have a real problem with excess accumulation of drugs in elderly patients.

These changes in adipose tissue help to explain a common clinical phenomenon in treating elderly patients with benzodiazepines. When starting benzos for anxiety or insomnia in the elderly, you might find that these patients don't respond to the very tiny doses with which we are taught to start. This is because the first few doses are whisked away into the patients' fat, rendering the medication less available and causing it to have a briefer duration of effect. However, with repeated dosing, the fat stores get saturated and benzo levels build up, so that a couple of weeks after starting treatment, these patients may develop signs of benzo toxicity such as sedation, cognitive impairment, and balance problems. Moreover, if you reduce or stop the medication, its excretion can take a very long time.

A more rational approach to this scenario is to "start normal, then reduce the dose," rather than "start low, go slow." This same argument could be applied to obese patients, although there tends to be less accumulation in younger patients because their liver and kidney functions are more robust.

While fat cells pull some drugs out of the bloodstream in the elderly, the brain also has a greater pull as people age because the blood-brain barrier becomes more permeable. This mainly affects lithium, as older patients do not need as much lithium in their bloodstream to achieve adequate levels in the CNS (see Chapter 9 and Chapter 12).

Biotransformation

All things deteriorate with age, livers and kidneys as much as car engines and roof shingles. Recall that most of the biotransformation of drugs occurs in the liver. As we age, the blood flow to the liver decreases, so that by age 65 there is 45% less blood coursing through the liver than at age 25. While this certainly causes some cell death, the liver was cleverly engineered with a redundancy of hepatocytes to ensure that it can continue to function pretty well into old age.

However, the decreased blood flow to the liver does affect first-pass metabolism, which is the step where drugs are transported to the liver from the intestine. The liver immediately extracts and deactivates a certain percentage of those molecules. If only half as much blood gets to the liver, a lower proportion of the drug will be extracted, leading to a higher spike in drug serum levels. Many psychotropics, including most antidepressants and antipsychotics, are affected by this change because 50% of their dose is deactivated by the liver on first pass. As hepatic blood flow falls with age, these medications will peak at higher serum concentration than normal. Benzodiazepines are less vulnerable to this change because only 10%–20% of their total dose is deactivated by the liver on first pass.

In addition to decreased hepatic blood flow, some of the CYP450 enzymes become sluggish in the elderly. Most notably for psychiatry, the 3A4 system slows down. Happily, the 2D6 system that metabolizes many psychotropics is less affected by age. Likewise, metabolism through the glucuronidation system (sometimes called Phase II metabolism) is not affected by age at all. This is why benzodiazepines that are metabolized through glucuronidation are often preferred in the elderly (lorazepam, oxazepam, and temazepam).

Excretion and the Aging Kidneys

On average, renal mass declines by 45% by age 80, and there are corresponding declines in renal function. Despite this glum statistic, about a third of the healthy elderly maintain essentially normal kidney function. Still, that leaves a substantial majority with renal impairment. But does it matter?

Reductions in kidney function are mainly relevant for the few psychiatric drugs that are metabolized primarily by the kidneys, especially lithium, gabapentin, pregabalin, and paliperidone (see Chapter 9). Those drugs will have higher serum levels and longer half-lives if the kidneys are slowed down. But there are other changes that tend to follow renal impairment—like reductions in protein binding and protein distribution—that can also affect medications metabolized through the liver. So, exercise caution (use lower doses and monitor more closely) even with drugs that are metabolized through the liver, particularly drugs that are highly protein bound and those with higher likelihoods of toxicity, longer half-lives, or active metabolites* that could accumulate when the kidneys are impaired.

How does one tell if a patient has impaired renal function? Significant renal disease will show up as elevations in the standard renal blood test—the creatinine level. But what about the healthy elderly patient without frank renal disease? Renal function tends to decline with age, but you can't detect this milder slowing by ordering a creatinine level. Creatinine is a byproduct of muscle tissue, and muscle mass decreases in the elderly. The reduction in creatinine clearance is offset by the decreased production of creatinine, which is why creatinine is not a reliable indicator here.

There is a way of measuring the kidneys' specific ability to clear creatinine, called the creatinine clearance test, but this involves collecting a patient's urine for 24 hours, a cumbersome process that most patients refuse unless absolutely necessary. However, there is a way to approximate creatinine clearance from serum creatinine by using the following formula, which takes into account the patient's age, weight, and blood creatinine level (for women, multiply the result by 0.85):

$$\text{Creatinine clearance} = \frac{(140 - \text{age in years}) \times (\text{body weight in kg})}{72 \times \text{serum creatinine level}}$$

You might be wondering if all this is more information than you really need to know as a psychiatrist. It may well be. The only time you would

---

*Psychotropics with active metabolites include antidepressants (citalopram, escitalopram, fluoxetine, sertraline; bupropion, mirtazapine, nefazodone, trazodone, venlafaxine; tranylcypromine, selegiline; amitriptyline, clomipramine, doxepin, imipramine); antipsychotics (aripiprazole, clozapine, loxapine, risperidone, quetiapine); anticonvulsants (carbamazepine, oxcarbazepine, valproate); sedatives (chlordiazepoxide, clorazepate, diazepam; doxepin, eszopiclone, and lemborexant); and the VMAT-2 inhibitor valbenazine.

try to estimate the creatinine clearance is when you can't figure out why a patient's serum lithium level is very high in the presence of a very low dose. But chances are you would refer such a patient to their primary care physician for a complete workup.

Protein Binding

What about protein binding and the elderly? In the absence of malnutrition or chronic GI problems, serum protein levels are not typically decreased in the elderly. And as we discussed in Chapter 10, drug interactions involving protein binding are generally not significant because any excess free fraction of a medication gets metabolized via normal routes. However, if your elderly patient has impaired hepatic metabolism, protein-binding interactions could result in sustained high serum levels of certain drugs.

The Bottom Line: How Should You Dose Drugs in the Elderly?

The effects of aging on drug metabolism are complicated. Some factors act to increase serum levels, such as decreased hepatic first-pass extraction, decreased CYP450 activity, and decreased renal clearance. Other factors can lower serum levels, such as a higher volume of distribution from adipose tissue. Add to this the unpredictable intra-individual variation in each patient's biology and you have a very confusing situation on your hands.

Thus, ultimately, the tried-and-true dictum applies in prescribing for the elderly: "Start low, go slow." While this won't be true for all patients or for all drugs (for example, "start normal, then reduce the dose" may apply to benzodiazepines) you have little to lose by hewing to this practice, whereas you can easily cause catastrophic outcomes with too-aggressive dosing.

What does "start low, go slow" mean in actual practice? A good rule is to start at half the standard adult dose and to titrate upwards at half your standard rate.

So far we've talked about pharmacokinetic changes in the elderly that influence how we dose medications. But pharmacodynamics change as patients age as well, making them more vulnerable to medications that cause orthostasis, QTc prolongation, temperature imbalance, falls, and anticholinergic effects, to name a few. A good resource to help you steer clear of those risks is the American Geriatrics Society, which keeps a list of medications that warrant caution in the elderly in their handy Beers

Criteria (American Geriatrics Society Beers Criteria® Update Expert Panel, *J Am Geriatr Soc* 2019;67(4):674–694).

Drug Metabolism in the Young

Our focus in this section will be on the toddler age group and above, because few psychiatrists are prescribing drugs for infants. This simplifies the job considerably, because most of the really complicated differences in drug metabolism occur only in the very very young.

The bottom line in prescribing for children is that you have to decrease doses of most psychiatric drugs in proportion to the lower weight of a given pediatric patient. This may not be a big news flash to most prescribers, but it isn't necessarily obvious, because some of us may well wonder whether a child's young and supple metabolic machinery might chew up drugs faster to compensate for their lower weight. In general, this isn't true, though there are some exceptions, so read on.

Absorption

A child's GI tract absorbs drugs similarly to that of an adult, but the transit through the GI tract tends to be shorter in children, particularly those under age 8. This may reduce the absorption of modified-release medications. For example, modified-release theophylline is more unpredictably absorbed in children than in adults. The implication is that modified-release stimulants like Adderall XR and Concerta might pass through a young child's GI tract too quickly to allow absorption of every last anti-ADHD molecule, resulting in a shorter duration of effect. You can compensate for such problems by increasing the dose or switching to an immediate-release form of the medication.

Biotransformation and Excretion

Children and adults share the same collection of metabolic enzymes, but the hepatic CYP enzymes are a bit faster in children, at least until adolescence. Similarly, renal filtration is faster in children. Both of these factors mean that, at least for some kids and for some drugs, dosing ends up being higher than what might be expected based on weight alone.

The main example of this is lithium. In studies of lithium in children (ages 6–12), doses up to 1500 mg/day were often required to reach adequate serum lithium levels. However, the target serum levels for lithium are the same for children as they are for adults (see Table 12-4, page 123). It's possible that children may also need higher doses of other renally cleared medications like gabapentin and pregabalin.

By adolescence, drug metabolism slows way down and approaches normal adult levels. Thus if you follow a patient from childhood into adolescence, you may actually need to decrease the dose of medication as the child becomes a teenager.

Prescribing for people at the outer age ranges is more complicated than what we can fit in this chapter. If you feel out of your zone of competence, it is often a good idea to consult with child and geriatric psychiatric colleagues who spend their careers in those spaces.

CHAPTER 19

Women, Men, and Medications

WE DON'T KNOW A LOT about gender and drug metabolism because women were often excluded from drug trials before the 1990s. The reasons ranged from the quasi-scientific ("Hormonal fluctuations will introduce too many variables into a clinical trial"); to the misogynistic ("The normal subject is the Caucasian male"); to the paternalistic, as in 1977 when the FDA banned women of childbearing age from participating in clinical trials to eliminate the risk of drug exposure in pregnancy. That 1977 rule was reversed in 1993 after women took on more leadership roles in medicine.

Psychopharmacology might have taken some different turns if more women had been included in the early trials. For example, we might have concluded that MAOIs are more effective than tricyclics because women respond better to this class of antidepressant.

Even less is known about pharmacokinetic differences in the way that women and men metabolize medications. Some hepatic enzymes are faster in women (CYP2D6, 2B6, and 3A4), while CYP1A2 is faster in men. These differences are small, however, and unlikely to have a clinical impact, with some exceptions such as zolpidem (Ambien).

Zolpidem: Different Doses for Different Genders

In 2013, zolpidem became the first psychiatric medication to include separate dosage recommendations for women and men. The FDA cut the maximum dose for women in half, from 10 mg to 5 mg, or to 6.25 mg if they are taking the CR version. Those guidelines are a bit on the conservative side, since zolpidem's clearance is only 35% lower in women than men, not 50%. Still, there's good reason to stick with those gender-based guidelines, as problems like falls, amnestic behaviors (including "complex sleep behaviors" like cooking in the middle of the night), and car accidents go up at higher serum levels.

Body mass explains part of this gender effect, but that only accounts for a third of the difference. The rest is probably related to the well-known difference in alcohol metabolism between women and men. In men, testosterone speeds up the enzymes responsible for alcohol's metabolism, alcohol and aldehyde dehydrogenase, and those enzymes are involved in the breakdown of zolpidem as well (Peer CJ et al, *Front Pharmacol* 2016;7:260). The result is that women metabolize alcohol, and zolpidem, slower than men. This testosterone effect is not known to occur with other z-hypnotics like zaleplon (Sonata) and eszopiclone (Lunesta), but differences in body mass may still make those hypnotics a little more potent in women than they are in men.

VERDICT

Keep zolpidem at 5 mg in women (or 6.25 mg if using the CR). The risks of going higher are rare but serious.

Serotonin

Women are more likely to have atypical symptoms of depression, such as overeating, oversleeping, rejection sensitivity, and heavy sensations in their limbs (leaden paralysis). That difference disappears after menopause. The reason this matters is that atypical depression responds better to MAOIs and SSRIs than to tricyclics. That may explain why some studies have found a gender-based difference in antidepressant response, favoring MAOIs and SSRIs in women, but there is more to this story.

When investigators adjusted for the higher rate of atypical symptoms in women, they found this gender difference in antidepressant response still held up (Keers R and Aitchison KJ, *Int Rev Psychiatry* 2010;22(5):485–500). So what explains the difference? One possibility is estrogen. Estrogen influences serotonergic transmission, and MAOIs and SSRIs depend on this monoamine for their therapeutic effects. Whatever the reason, this gender-based difference is mild and is not a reason to avoid tricyclics in women.

Serotonin receptors become more sensitive when estrogen levels fall in the week or two before menses, which can make some women feel like their SSRI is not working during that period. One solution is to raise the dose of the SSRI 2 weeks before menses, usually doubling it.

A similar strategy is used for premenstrual dysphoric disorder, which can be treated by taking an SSRI for the 2 weeks before menses and holding it for the other half of the month. In 2000, fluoxetine became the first SSRI approved for this use, as the pink-and-purple Sarafem capsule. Sertraline and paroxetine are also approved in premenstrual dysphoric disorder, but fluoxetine is a good one to start with because its long half-life reduces the risk that this on/off dosing will cause withdrawal problems.

VERDICT

Women tend to respond better to SSRIs and MAOIs than tricyclics, while men show the opposite pattern, but the differences are slight. Some women who take serotonergic antidepressants may need to raise the dose in the 2 weeks before their menstrual cycle.

Side Effects

Side effects also differ between the sexes. Women are more likely to experience weight gain, hyperglycemia, and cardiac arrhythmias, while men have to worry more about priapism with trazodone (although this painful erection can happen to the clitoris as well). Women are more likely to experience sexual dysfunction on psychiatric medications, but the rates are pretty high for both genders. Phosphodiesterase-5 inhibitors like sildenafil (Viagra) are among the best-studied antidotes for sexual dysfunction on antidepressants, and surprisingly their benefits extend to both women and men (Nurnberg HG et al, *JAMA* 2008;300(4):395–404). These medications improve blood flow to the penis and clitoris, and they have CNS effects as well, enhancing dopaminergic transmission in areas of the brain involved in sexual arousal (Kyratsas C et al, *J Sex Med* 2013;10(3):719–729).

Duloxetine has a particular side effect that can play out differently in women and men. This antidepressant tightens the sphincter in the bladder, which is a good thing if your patient has stress incontinence, a problem that is 4 times more common in women than men. But a tight sphincter can also cause urine retention, something that men are more vulnerable to as they age and their prostate enlarges. Surprisingly, another SNRI—venlafaxine—can have the opposite effect of causing urine incontinence.

Other medical risks that differ between women and men are listed in tables 19-1 and 19-2 and summarized in the Verdict below.

VERDICT

Medications that cause problems in women include full-dose zolpidem (10–12.5 mg), valproate, prolactin-raising antipsychotics, and, in postmenopausal women at risk for osteoporosis, serotonergic antidepressants. Side effects to watch for in men include priapism and ejaculatory dysfunction. Both men and women can benefit from phosphodiesterase-5 inhibitors for sexual dysfunction on SSRIs.

**TABLE 19-1. Medical Risks With Psychotropics
That Are More Likely in Women**

Osteoporosis	Bone mineral loss can occur in postmenopausal women on: Serotonergic antidepressants Antipsychotics that raise prolactin Carbamazepine Thyroid augmentation in depression
Breast cancer	Antipsychotics that raise prolactin
Polycystic ovarian disease	Valproic acid
Urinary incontinence	Risperidone, olanzapine, clozapine, gabapentin, SSRIs, venlafaxine, prazosin, and sedatives

**TABLE 19-2. Medical Risks With Psychotropics
That Are More Likely in Men**

Priapism	Trazodone
Ejaculatory dysfunction	Antipsychotics
Urinary retention	MAOIs, alpha-adrenoceptor agonists (clonidine, guanfacine), phenothiazine, antipsychotics, antihistamines, anticholinergics, and opiates

Drugs of Abuse

The medical consequences of drug abuse are generally worse for women than men. Women clear alcohol more slowly. They are less likely to benefit from the purportedly positive effects of low-dose drinking and more likely to develop cancer (especially breast cancer), liver disease, and heart disease as their alcohol intake goes up. Women clear nicotine more rapidly than men, but that doesn't clear the carcinogenic hydrocarbons in the smoke. Women are 20%–70% more likely to get lung cancer from smoking than men even when they smoke the same number of cigarettes.

Women are also more likely to be victims of abuse when intoxicated, including involuntary intoxication through drugs that we prescribe, like benzodiazepines and z-hypnotics. Some of the most notorious offenders are now highly restricted and rarely prescribed because of their reputation as "date rape" drugs, including flunitrazepam (Rohypnol, "roofies"), gamma-hydroxybutyrate (Xyrem), chloral hydrate, and ketamine.

CHAPTER 20

Drug Metabolism and Ethnicity

NO DOUBT, PATIENTS DIFFER IN their genes, environment, and culture. Ethnicity is a rough way of categorizing these differences at best, and a source of prejudice and misunderstanding at worst. Non-Caucasian populations have suffered from significant disparities in access to psychiatric and mental health care. They have experienced race-related differences in diagnosis, treatment, and outcomes, as well as participation in research. With those limitations in mind, we'll present here four ways that biological response to medications may differ among ethnic groups.

Drug Metabolism

Some populations have higher rates of poor metabolism in the CYP enzymes. Their metabolic enzymes are very slow or blocked, resulting in higher serum levels and more side effects, as well as unexpected efficacy in the lower dose range.

Around 20%–40% of Asians from China, Korea, and Japan are poor metabolizers at pathways that are important in psychiatry—CYP2D6, CYP3A4, or CYP2C19—rates that are 2–4 times higher than those seen in Caucasians. This may explain why clinical trials in East Asian populations generally arrive at doses that are 30%–50% below those used in Caucasian populations when the researchers are allowed to flexibly dose the medication based on response.

Hispanics and African Americans have high rates of both poor and rapid metabolism, depending on their country of origin. In practice, this generally translates to higher rates of side effects with poor metabolizers and lack of efficacy with rapid metabolizers (Henderson DC and Vincenzi B. Ethnopsychopharmacology. In: Lim RF, ed. *Clinical Manual of Cultural Psychiatry*. 2nd ed. Arlington, VA: American Psychiatric Publishing; 2015:435–468).

Around 1 in 3 Asian patients require lower doses of medications that pass through the CYP system. For Caucasians, that rate is closer to 1 in 10. Among Hispanics and African Americans, expect a lot more variety, with higher rates of both poor and rapid metabolizers.

Pharmacogenetic Testing and the SERT Gene

Pharmacogenetic testing can clarify the metabolic differences among ethnic populations (see Chapter 17), but those tests are not very reliable when it comes to pharmacodynamic genes that predict drug response. Ethnicity may partly explain why.

Individual genes act very differently in the brain depending on the environment and the other genes they are paired with, just as the color blue is perceived differently depending on the lighting that surrounds it and whether you mix it with a little yellow paint. We see this play out with one of the most popular genetic tests—the serotonin transporter (SERT) gene, which is supposed to predict response to SSRIs.

In theory, a short (S) SERT allele is thought to predict a poor response to SSRIs, while a long (L) allele suggests a more favorable course. However, that finding has only held up among Caucasian men. In Asian populations we see the opposite trend, with the short arm predicting a slightly more favorable response to SSRIs (Bousman CA et al, *J Clin Psychopharmacol* 2014;34(5):645–648). The frequency of this short allele also varies by ethnicity: 50% in Caucasians, 30% in Africans, and 70% in Asians (Gelernter J et al, *Hum Genet* 1997;101(2):243–246).

VERDICT
Although marketed to predict SSRI response, the SERT gene does this reliably in only one ethnic minority: the Caucasian male (who comprises 30% of the US and 10% of the global population). Even there, its predictive value is nowhere near 100%.

Adverse Effects

Some adverse effects occur more frequently in certain ethnic groups even at normal drug levels. Asians are 10 times more likely to develop severe allergic rashes with carbamazepine. You can test for this risk with HLA genotyping, and the FDA now requires that test before prescribing carbamazepine to patients of Asian descent (see "Genes for Drug Allergies" on page 173).

The antipsychotics are another area where we see strong ethnic differences in response. Asians are more prone to hyperprolactinemia, while African Americans are more vulnerable to metabolic and cardiac side effects on these drugs (Lin KM, *J Clin Psychopharmacol* 1988;8(3):195–201). One reviewer found that nearly half of the published case reports of new-onset diabetes on atypical antipsychotics occurred in African Americans (Jin H et al, *Ann Clin Psychiatry* 2002;14(1):59–64). Extrapyramidal symptoms are more common in Asians, Hispanics, and African Americans, and African Americans are more likely to develop tardive dyskinesia.

Clozapine and Benign Neutropenia in African Americans

Certain ethnic groups have lower than average absolute neutrophil counts (ANC). This condition, benign ethnic neutropenia (BEN), is a normal finding and not a reason to avoid or discontinue clozapine therapy. BEN is more common in persons of African descent (25%–50%), some Middle Eastern ethnic groups (Yemenite Jews, Jordanians), and other non-Caucasian ethnic groups with darker skin (Rajagopal S, *Postgrad Med* 2005;81(959):545–546). A hematology consultation can clarify if a patient's low ANC is due to BEN, and the clozapine guidelines have separate standards for identifying agranulocytosis in the context of BEN (see www.clozapinerems.com). While BEN is more common in male African Americans, genuine clozapine-induced agranulocytosis occurs more often in women and in patients of Asian or Ashkenazi Jewish descent (Rajagopal, 2005).

VERDICT

Don't pass on clozapine just because your patient has a low white blood count. If they are African American, Middle Eastern, or from another darker-skinned race, refer to a hematologist to rule out BEN. For Asian patients, always check the HLA-B*1502 gene before starting carbamazepine. It's required for that drug, and probably a good idea for oxcarbazepine as well.

Tables of Relevant Drug Interactions

WHEN YOUR ONLY TASK IS to look up an interaction between two or more specific drugs, computer software is perfectly adequate. But more often than not, this is not the kind of information you need while you're making medication decisions. Most of the time during psychopharm visits, you are sifting through a mental list of many candidate medications that you might use for a patient.

For example, in the case of patients with comorbid anxiety and depression, you will typically be entertaining a list of 10 or 20 medications that might be helpful. Assuming that the patient is already taking two or three meds (psychiatric and nonpsychiatric), there will be dozens of possible interactions. As drug options pop into your mind, you don't want to have to enter each possible combination into a software drug interactions program, only to find a long list of "potential" interactions that may not be clinically significant. Instead, it is often more useful to have a couple of well-organized charts that lay all the information out graphically.

How to Use the Psychiatric Drug Interactions by Medication Chart

Most published drug interaction charts are categorized by P450 enzyme family rather than by medication. But we don't organize our clinical thinking in terms of 2D6s and 3A4s; instead, we think in terms of drug classes and specific members of those classes. Thus, a more useful chart is an alphabetical list of commonly used psychiatric medications, with information about how "clean" or "dirty" each one is in combination with other drugs. We've created this type of chart, **Psychiatric Drug Interactions by Medication,** on page 200.

Here's an example of how you can use this chart. Let's assume you have a patient on valproate for bipolar disorder. One day he comes into your office with racing thoughts and mild paranoia. Aside from reviewing his valproate level and considering a dosage increase, you decide to prescribe one of the atypical antipsychotics, all of which are FDA approved for treating manic episodes. But you want to avoid prescribing anything that will affect your patient's valproate level. You could pull out your smartphone and input valproate along with each of the several antipsychotics you might prescribe—or, you could quickly glance at the Psychiatric Drug Interactions by Medication chart under valproate and look at the "Red Flags" column. There you'll see that the only clinically relevant interaction is that valproate increases levels of lamotrigine—not an issue in this case, since your patient is not taking lamotrigine. Just to be sure, you can then look at the section of the chart on "Second-Generation Antipsychotics," and you'll see that only two of these medications cause significant drug interactions (asenapine and risperidone), but they inhibit CYP2D6, which valproate is not a substrate of. So, you're in the clear, and you can go ahead and prescribe your atypical of choice knowing that it will not mess with your patient's valproate levels.

How to Use the Psychiatric Drug Interactions by Enzyme Family Chart

While the chart organized by meds is helpful, it is not always sufficient—there are times when it is helpful to have a chart organized by enzyme family. This is particularly important when you need to know not only whether the drug you are prescribing will affect the levels of other drugs, but whether its own level will be altered by drugs that your patient is already taking. This is why the column in the Psychiatric Drug Interactions by Medication chart labeled "Substrate of" is important. It tells you what enzyme families are primarily responsible for metabolizing that medication. You then need to look up the relevant enzyme families to see what drugs affect them. For this, you want a drug interaction chart organized by enzyme families. Our version of this chart, **Psychiatric Drug Interactions by Enzyme Family,** is found on page 211.

Suppose that you have a patient with schizophrenia who has been maintained on quetiapine, but now is suffering major depression. He is already somewhat sedated on the quetiapine, so you want to make sure that whatever you prescribe will not increase his quetiapine levels. The

Psychiatric Drug Interactions by Medication chart tells you that quetiapine is metabolized primarily by 3A4, so you look at the list of antidepressants in the Psychiatric Drug Interactions by Enzyme Family chart to see if any of them inhibit 3A4. The only ones that do are fluvoxamine and nefazodone. You forgo those and prescribe sertraline.

A Few Tips on How to Use the "Carlat Charts" in Your Office

1. Just because an interaction is listed doesn't mean that it will necessarily cause clinical problems for your patient. According to most authorities, only 10%–20% of patients will be unlucky enough to develop clinical consequences when prescribed interacting drugs. But those are still high enough odds to be vigilant.

2. Focus on interactions involving drugs with the potential for serious toxicity. Among psychiatric drugs, some of the more potentially dangerous drugs include bupropion (seizure risk), clozapine (ileus, orthostasis, and arrythmias), lithium (confusion, ataxia), lamotrigine (rash risk), and a few that can cause cardiac arrythmias at high levels (tricyclics, citalopram, ziprasidone, pimozide, and the VMAT-2 inhibitors).

3. When starting a patient on a potent enzyme inhibitor, consider cutting the dose of a vulnerable drug in half right away, since inhibitory effects occur immediately.

4. When starting a patient on a potent enzyme inducer (such as carbamazepine), find out if she is on a drug that is vulnerable to induction (in the case of carbamazepine, a substrate of 3A4 or several other pathways). If so, wait about a week before increasing the dosage of that drug, because it takes inducers about that long to rev up the production of extra P450 enzymes.

5. When a medication is listed as being the substrate of multiple enzymes, chances are that no inhibiting drug will increase its level much, since if one enzyme is impaired, others can take over. (An exception to this rule is the tricyclics, whose metabolism is significantly inhibited by some SSRIs that inhibit several enzymes.) This moderating effect of multiple enzymes doesn't apply when the other drug is an inducer, however, because a single supercharged enzyme can chew up substrate quickly, even while other enzymes are sitting around and yawning.

6. Do you know your patient's metabolizer status? If they've had genetic testing done, you might. For example, if your patient is a slow

metabolizer, a moderate interaction can act like a strong one because the enzyme system is already slowed down.

To keep the charts practical, we've listed only the major pathways for drug metabolism, and only the inhibitors and inducers that have a strong effect on those pathways. For example, venlafaxine is a substrate of CYP2D6, 3A4, and 2C19, but 2D6 does the brunt of the work, so interactions that affect the other enzymes will not alter its levels much.

TABLE A-1. How to Adjust a Victim Drug

Type of Interaction	Dosage Adjustment
Strong inhibitor	Multiply target dose by 0.25–0.5
Moderate inhibitor	Multiply target dose by 0.7–0.8
Strong inducer	Multiply target dose by 2–4

TABLE A-2. Psychiatric Drug Interactions by Medication

Medication	Substrate of	Strongly Inhibits	Strongly Induces	Red Flags*
SSRI Antidepressants				
Citalopram (Celexa)^M	2C19, 3A4			Max dose 20 mg/day with 2C19 inhibitors like proton pump inhibitors due to QTc prolongation
Escitalopram (Lexapro)^M	2C19, 3A4			
Fluoxetine (Prozac)^M	2D6, 2C9	2D6, 2C19		Increases tricyclics, antipsychotics
Fluvoxamine (Luvox)	2D6, 1A2	1A2, 2C19		Increases clozapine, asenapine
Paroxetine (Paxil)	2D6	2D6, 2B6		Increases tricyclics, antipsychotics
Sertraline (Zoloft)^M	2C19	At ≥ 150 mg/day: 2D6		Increases tricyclics, antipsychotics

^M These medications are converted into active metabolites. In most cases the metabolites have similar effects as the parent drug, with the exception of nefazodone and trazodone (converted into mCPP, which can cause depression and anxiety if the levels rise too quickly), clozapine (converted into norclozapine, which adds to side effect burden), quetiapine (converted into norquetiapine, which has antidepressant properties), loxapine (converted into the tricyclic amoxapine), and eszopiclone (converted into the non-sedating anxiolytic desmethylzopiclone).

*Red flags identify potentially serious interactions. The list is not comprehensive.

(table continues)

TABLE A-2. Psychiatric Drug Interactions by Medication *(continued)*

Medication	Substrate of	Strongly Inhibits	Strongly Induces	Red Flags*
SNRI Antidepressants				
Desvenlafaxine (Pristiq)	UGT-1A1			
Duloxetine (Cymbalta)	1A2, 2D6	2D6		Increases tricyclics, antipsychotics
Levomilnacipran (Fetzima)	3A4			
Milnacipran (Savella)	UGTs			
Venlafaxine (Effexor)ᴹ	2D6			
Tricyclic Antidepressants				
Amitriptyline (Elavil)ᴹ	2D6, 2C19, 3A4, 1A2			Tricyclics are increased by various 2D6 inhibitors
Amoxapine (Asendin)	2D6			
Clomipramine (Anafranil)ᴹ	2D6, 2C19, 1A2	2D6		
Desipramine (Norpramin)	2D6			
Doxepin (Sinequan, Silenor)ᴹ	2D6, 2C19	2D6		
Imipramine (Tofranil)ᴹ	2D6, 2C19	2D6		
Maprotiline (Ludiomil)	2D6			
Nortriptyline (Pamelor)	2D6			
Protriptyline (Vivactil)	2D6			
Trimipramine (Surmontil)	2D6			

ᴹThese medications are converted into active metabolites. In most cases the metabolites have similar effects as the parent drug, with the exception of nefazodone and trazodone (converted into mCPP, which can cause depression and anxiety if the levels rise too quickly), clozapine (converted into norclozapine, which adds to side effect burden), quetiapine (converted into norquetiapine, which has antidepressant properties), loxapine (converted into the tricyclic amoxapine), and eszopiclone (converted into the nonsedating anxiolytic desmethylzopiclone).

*Red flags identify potentially serious interactions. The list is not comprehensive.

(table continues)

TABLE A-2. Psychiatric Drug Interactions by Medication *(continued)*

Medication	Substrate of	Strongly Inhibits	Strongly Induces	Red Flags*
MAOI Antidepressants				
Isocarboxazid (Marplan)	Non-CYP			Dietary and drug interactions (see pages 142 & 145)
Phenelzine (Nardil)	Non-CYP			
Selegiline patch (EMSAM)	2B6			
Tranylcypromine (Parnate)	2A6			
Other Antidepressants				
Bupropion (Wellbutrin)^M	2B6	2D6		Increases fluoxetine, fluvoxamine, paroxetine, venlafaxine, vortioxetine, tricyclics, and antipsychotics
Mirtazapine (Remeron)^M	1A2, 2D6, 3A4			
Nefazodone (Serzone)^M	3A4	3A4		Increases carbamazepine, guanfacine, modafinils, antipsychotics, benzos, and z-hypnotics
St. John's wort	Unclear		1A2, 2C9, 2C19, 3A4	Decreases OCPs and multiple medications
Trazodone (Desyrel)^M	3A4			
Vilazodone (Viibryd)	3A4			
Vortioxetine (Trintellix)	2D6, 3A4, 3A5			Levels doubled by bupropion and possibly other 2D6 inhibitors

^MThese medications are converted into active metabolites. In most cases the metabolites have similar effects as the parent drug, with the exception of nefazodone and trazodone (converted into mCPP, which can cause depression and anxiety if the levels rise too quickly), clozapine (converted into norclozapine, which adds to side effect burden), quetiapine (converted into norquetiapine, which has antidepressant properties), loxapine (converted into the tricyclic amoxapine), and eszopiclone (converted into the non-sedating anxiolytic desmethylzopiclone).

*Red flags identify potentially serious interactions. The list is not comprehensive.

(table continues)

TABLE A-2. Psychiatric Drug Interactions by Medication *(continued)*

Medication	Substrate of	Strongly Inhibits	Strongly Induces	Red Flags*
Mood Stabilizers				
Carbamazepine (Tegretol, Equetro)^M	3A4		1A2, 3A4, 2C8, 2C9, 2C19, 2B6, UGT-1A4	Decreases OCPs, lamotrigine, and many others (see page 121)
Lamotrigine (Lamictal)	UGT-1A4			Increased by valproate; decreased by estrogen and carbamazepine
Lithium (Lithobid, Eskalith)	Renal (excreted unchanged)			Increased by NSAIDs, ACE inhibitors, diuretics
Valproate (Depakote)^M	UGTs (1A6, 1A9, 2B7), 2C9, 2A6, 2B6, 3A5	UGTs (1A4, 1A9, 2B7, 2B15), 2C9		Doubles lamotrigine levels
Other Anticonvulsants				
Gabapentin (Neurontin)	Renal (excreted unchanged)			
Levetiracetam (Keppra)	Mainly renal (66% excreted unchanged)			
Oxcarbazepine (Trileptal)^M	UGT	2C19	3A4, UGT-1A4 at ≥ 1200 mg	At ≥ 1200 mg, lowers multiple medications including OCPs (effect is 50% that of carbamazepine)
Pregabalin (Lyrica)	Renal (excreted unchanged)			
Tiagabine (Gabitril)	3A4			
Topiramate (Topamax)	Mainly renal (70% excreted unchanged)		2C19, 3A4 at ≥ 200 mg	Decreases OCPs at ≥ 200 mg; decreased 50% by carbamazepine
Zonisamide (Zonegran)	3A4			

^MThese medications are converted into active metabolites. In most cases the metabolites have similar effects as the parent drug, with the exception of nefazodone and trazodone (converted into mCPP, which can cause depression and anxiety if the levels rise too quickly), clozapine (converted into norclozapine, which adds to side effect burden), quetiapine (converted into norquetiapine, which has antidepressant properties), loxapine (converted into the tricyclic amoxapine), and eszopiclone (converted into the non-sedating anxiolytic desmethylzopiclone).

*Red flags identify potentially serious interactions. The list is not comprehensive.

(table continues)

TABLE A-2. Psychiatric Drug Interactions by Medication *(continued)*

Medication	Substrate of	Strongly Inhibits	Strongly Induces	Red Flags*
Second-Generation Antipsychotics				
Aripiprazole (Abilify)^M	2D6, 3A4			
Asenapine (Saphris, Secuado)	1A2, UGT-1A4	2D6		Increases antidepressants. It is the antipsychotic least likely to interact with carbamazepine.
Brexpiprazole (Rexulti)	2D6, 3A4			
Cariprazine (Vraylar)	3A4			
Clozapine (Clozaril)^M	1A2			
Iloperidone (Fanapt)	2D6, 3A4			
Lumateperone (Caplyta)	3A4			
Lurasidone (Latuda)	3A4			
Olanzapine (Zyprexa)	1A2, UGT-1A4			
Paliperidone (Invega)	Renal (primarily excreted unchanged)			Levels decreased 40%–70% by carbamazepine and increased 50% by valproate through changes in renal clearance
Pimavanserin (Nuplazid)	3A4			
Quetiapine (Seroquel)^M	3A4			
Risperidone (Risperdal)^M	2D6	2D6		
Ziprasidone (Geodon)	3A4			

^M These medications are converted into active metabolites. In most cases the metabolites have similar effects as the parent drug, with the exception of nefazodone and trazodone (converted into mCPP, which can cause depression and anxiety if the levels rise too quickly), clozapine (converted into norclozapine, which adds to side effect burden), quetiapine (converted into norquetiapine, which has antidepressant properties), loxapine (converted into the tricyclic amoxapine), and eszopiclone (converted into the non-sedating anxiolytic desmethylzopiclone).

*Red flags identify potentially serious interactions. The list is not comprehensive.

(table continues)

TABLE A-2. Psychiatric Drug Interactions by Medication *(continued)*

Medication	Substrate of	Strongly Inhibits	Strongly Induces	Red Flags*
First-Generation Antipsychotics				
Chlorpromazine (Thorazine)	2D6			
Fluphenazine (Prolixin)	2D6			
Haloperidol (Haldol)	2D6, 3A4	2D6		
Loxapine (Loxitane)^M	2D6, 3A4, 1A2			
Perphenazine (Trilafon)	2D6	2D6		
Pimozide (Orap)	2D6, 3A4, 1A2			Avoid with 2D6, 3A4, and 1A2 inhibitors as high levels can prolong QTc
Thioridazine (Mellaril)	2D6			
Thiothixene (Navane)	1A2			
Trifluoperazine (Stelazine)	1A2			
Stimulants and ADHD Medications				
Amphetamines (Adderall, Vyvanse, etc)	2D6 and other complex pathways			
Methylphenidates (Ritalin, Concerta, Focalin, etc)	2D6 and other complex pathways			
Atomoxetine (Strattera)	2D6			QTc prolongation with 2D6 inhibitors
Clonidine (Kapvay)	50% renal and 50% CYP (2D6, 1A2, 3A4, 1A1, 3A5)			
Guanfacine (Intuniv)	3A4			Hypotension with 3A4 inhibitors
Modafinil (Provigil), Armodafinil (Nuvigil)	3A4		3A4	May decrease OCPs
Viloxazine (Qelbree)	2D6, UGTs (1A9, 2B15)	1A2		

^M These medications are converted into active metabolites. In most cases the metabolites have similar effects as the parent drug, with the exception of nefazodone and trazodone (converted into mCPP, which can cause depression and anxiety if the levels rise too quickly), clozapine (converted into norclozapine, which adds to side effect burden), quetiapine (converted into norquetiapine, which has antidepressant properties), loxapine (converted into the tricyclic amoxapine), and eszopiclone (converted into the non-sedating anxiolytic desmethylzopiclone).

*Red flags identify potentially serious interactions. The list is not comprehensive.

(table continues)

TABLE A-2. Psychiatric Drug Interactions by Medication (continued)

Medication	Substrate of	Strongly Inhibits	Strongly Induces	Red Flags*
Addiction Medications				
Acamprosate (Campral)	Renal (excreted unchanged)			
Buprenorphine (Suboxone ingredient)	3A4			Increased by nefazodone, decreased by carbamazepine
Disulfiram (Antabuse)	Unknown	2E1		Hangover effects possible with small amounts of alcohol, including swallowed mouthwash or inhaled hand sanitizer
Lofexidine (Lucemyra)	2D6			Bradycardia, hypotension with 2D6 inhibitors
Methadone (Methadose, Dolophine)	3A4			Increased by nefazodone, decreased by carbamazepine
Naltrexone (ReVia, Vivitrol)	UGTs (2B7, 1A1, and other non-CYP)			Blocks opioids and can precipitate their withdrawal
Varenicline (Chantix)	Renal (90% excreted unchanged)			

*Red flags identify potentially serious interactions. The list is not comprehensive.

(table continues)

TABLE A-2. Psychiatric Drug Interactions by Medication *(continued)*

Medication	Substrate of	Strongly Inhibits	Strongly Induces	Red Flags*
Benzodiazepines				
Alprazolam (Xanax)	3A4			Strong 3A4 inhibitors (nefazodone and fluvoxamine) increase benzo levels. Strong 3A4 inducers (carbamazepine) decrease benzo levels. Benzos metabolized through UGT are usually free of interactions, but valproate doubles lorazepam levels.
Chlordiazepoxide (Librium)ᴹ	3A4			
Clonazepam (Klonopin)	3A4			
Clorazepate (Tranxene)ᴹ	3A4			
Diazepam (Valium)ᴹ	2C19, 3A4			
Estazolam (Prosom)	3A4			
Flurazepam (Dalmane)	3A4			
Lorazepam (Ativan)	UGT-2B7			
Oxazepam (Serax)	UGTs (2B15, 1A9, 2B7)			
Quazepam (Doral)	3A4, 2C9			
Temazepam (Restoril)	UGT-2B7			
Triazolam (Halcion)	3A4			
Hypnotics				
Doxepin (Silenor)ᴹ	2D6, 2C19	2D6		Strong 3A4 inhibitors double levels of z-hypnotics (eg, nefazodone), while inducers lower them (eg, carbamazepine). Ramelteon is raised by 1A2 inhibitors (eg, fluvoxamine).
Eszopiclone (Lunesta)ᴹ	3A4, 2E1			
Lemborexant (Dayvigo)ᴹ	3A4			
Melatonin	1A2			
Ramelteon (Rozerem)	1A2			
Suvorexant (Belsomra)	3A4			
Tasimelteon (Hetlioz)	3A4, 1A2			
Zaleplon (Sonata)	3A4			
Zolpidem (Ambien)	3A4			

ᴹThese medications are converted into active metabolites. In most cases the metabolites have similar effects as the parent drug, with the exception of nefazodone and trazodone (converted into mCPP, which can cause depression and anxiety if the levels rise too quickly), clozapine (converted into norclozapine, which adds to side effect burden), quetiapine (converted into norquetiapine, which has antidepressant properties), loxapine (converted into the tricyclic amoxapine), and eszopiclone (converted into the non-sedating anxiolytic desmethylzopiclone).

*Red flags identify potentially serious interactions. The list is not comprehensive.

(table continues)

TABLE A-2. Psychiatric Drug Interactions by Medication (continued)

Medication	Substrate of	Strongly Inhibits	Strongly Induces	Red Flags*
Dementia Medications				
Donepezil (Aricept)	2D6, 3A4			Caution with anticholinergics and beta blockers
Galantamine (Razadyne)	50% excreted unchanged in urine, 50% through 2D6, 3A4, and UGTs			
Memantine (Namenda)	Renal (75% excreted unchanged in urine)			
Rivastigmine (Exelon)	Renal and cholinesterases			
Sexual Dysfunction Medications				
Bremelanotide (Vyleesi)	Non-CYP			
Flibanserin (Addyi)	3A4			Syncope with 3A4 inhibitors (eg, fluvoxamine)
PDE5 inhibitors: avanafil (Stendra), sildenafil (Viagra), tadalafil (Cialis), vardenafil (Levitra)	3A4			Contraindicated with nitrates and alpha blockers (eg, prazosin)
Others				
Benztropine (Cogentin)	2D6 and non-CYP			
Buspirone (Buspar)	3A4			
Caffeine	1A2			
Cannabidiol (CBD oil)	3A4, 2C19	2D6 and possibly others		May raise tricyclics, antidepressants, antipsychotics, VMAT-2 inhibitors

*Red flags identify potentially serious interactions. The list is not comprehensive.

(table continues)

TABLE A-2. Psychiatric Drug Interactions by Medication *(continued)*

Medication	Substrate of	Strongly Inhibits	Strongly Induces	Red Flags*
Curcumin (Turmeric)		3A4		May raise opioids, benzos, and z-hypnotics
Deutetrabenazine (Austedo)	2D6			QTc prolongation with inhibitors
Dextromethorphan (in Nuedexta)	2D6, 3A4			
Esketamine (Spravato)	3A4, 2B6			
Grapefruit juice		3A4		Increases multiple medications (see page 129)
Nicotine	2A6, 2B6, UGT-2B10			
Ondansetron	3A4			
Pramipexole (Mirapex)	Renal (excreted unchanged)			
Propranolol (Inderal)	2D6			Bradycardia, hypotension at high levels
Quinidine (in Nuedexta)	3A4	2D6		Quinidine is in Nuedexta because the 2D6 inhibitor prolongs the half-life of the active ingredient, dextromethorphan. It also raises tricyclics, antidepressants, antipsychotics, and VMAT-2 inhibitors.
Samidorphan (in Lybalvi)	3A4			Blocks opioids and can precipitate their withdrawal

*Red flags identify potentially serious interactions. The list is not comprehensive.

(table continues)

TABLE A-2. Psychiatric Drug Interactions by Medication *(continued)*

Medication	Substrate of	Strongly Inhibits	Strongly Induces	Red Flags*
Smoking (hydrocarbons)			1A2	Decreases clozapine, haloperidol, olanzapine, and others: duloxetine, fluvoxamine, mirtazapine, propranolol, ramelteon
Testosterone	2B6, 3A4			
Valbenazine (Ingrezza)^M	2D6, 3A4			QTc prolongation with inhibitors

^{M}These medications are converted into active metabolites. In most cases the metabolites have similar effects as the parent drug, with the exception of nefazodone and trazodone (converted into mCPP, which can cause depression and anxiety if the levels rise too quickly), clozapine (converted into norclozapine, which adds to side effect burden), quetiapine (converted into norquetiapine, which has antidepressant properties), loxapine (converted into the tricyclic amoxapine), and eszopiclone (converted into the non-sedating anxiolytic desmethylzopiclone).

*Red flags identify potentially serious interactions. The list is not comprehensive.

TABLE A-3. Psychiatric Drug Interactions by Enzyme Family

P450 Family	Inhibitors	Inducers	Substrates	
			Psychiatric	Nonpsychiatric
3A4	**Grapefruit juice** Fluoxetine Fluvoxamine **Nefazodone** Paroxetine Sertraline (≥ 150 mg/day)	**Carbamazepine** Modafinils Oxcarbazepine (≥ 1200 mg/day) **St. John's wort** Topiramate (≥ 200 mg/day)	**Buspirone** (Inh: N/V, dizziness, sedation) **Carbamazepine** (Inh: fatigue, confusion; Ind: breakthrough seizures) **Citalopram** (Inh: arrhythmias) **Guanfacine** (Inh: hypotension) **Hypnotics, benzos** (Inh: sedation, falls, cognitive problems; Ind: lack of efficacy) **Methadone** (Inh: sedation, miosis; Ind: opioid withdrawal) **Modafinils** (Inh: insomnia, anxiety) **Tricyclics** (Inh: sedation, arrhythmias) **Valbenazine** (Inh: arrhythmias)	**Birth control pills** (Ind: pregnancy) **Calcium channel blockers** (Inh: hypotension) **Cyclosporine** (Ind: transplant rejection) **Statins** (Inh: ↑ LFTs, rhabdomyolysis) **Zonisamide, tiagabine** (Inh: seizures)
2D6	**Asenapine Bupropion Cannabidiol** Clozapine **Duloxetine** First-generation antipsychotics **Fluoxetine Paroxetine** Risperidone **Sertraline (≥ 150 mg/day)** Tricyclics	No inducers	**Antipsychotics Duloxetine Tricyclics** (Inh: sedation, arrhythmias) **Venlafaxine VMAT-2 inhibitors** (Inh: arrhythmias)	**Beta blockers** (Inh: hypotension) **Hydrocodone** (Inh: prodrug—less analgesia) **Tramadol** (Inh: prodrug—less analgesia)
1A2	**Fluvoxamine**	Cannabidiol **Carbamazepine** Melatonin Smoking **St. John's wort**	**Asenapine, clozapine, olanzapine, trifluoperazine, thiothixene Caffeine** (Inh: jittery) **Clozapine** (Inh: orthostasis, sedation) **Duloxetine Fluvoxamine Melatonin Ramelteon** (Inh: sedation)	None of great significance
2C9	Fluoxetine Fluvoxamine **St. John's wort** Valproate	**Carbamazepine**	None of great significance	**Oral hypoglycemics** (Inh: low blood sugar) Warfarin

Key: "Inh" = inhibition; "Ind" = induction; "N/V" = nausea/vomiting; "prodrug" means that the parent compound is metabolized into the active agent; in these cases, inhibition leads to less drug activity.
Strong inhibitors/inducers in bold. Moderate inhibitors/inducers in plain text.

(table continues)

TABLE A-3. Psychiatric Drug Interactions by Enzyme Family *(continued)*

P450 Family	Inhibitors	Inducers	Substrates	
			Psychiatric	Nonpsychiatric
2B6	Fluoxetine Fluvoxamine **Paroxetine** Sertraline (≥ 150 mg/day)	**Carbamazepine**	Bupropion Selegiline	None of great significance
2C19	**Fluoxetine Fluvoxamine** Oxcarbazepine Sertraline (≥ 150 mg/day)	**Carbamazepine St. John's wort**	Citalopram (Inh: arrhythmias) Escitalopram Sertraline Tricyclics	None of great significance
Protein binding	**Fluoxetine Paroxetine Prozac Sertraline Valproate**	No significant inducers	None of great significance	**Digoxin** (Inh: arrhythmia, N/V, confusion) **Phenytoin** (Inh: confusion, ataxia) **Warfarin** (Inh: ↑ PT, bruising, bleeding)

Key: "Inh" = inhibition; "Ind" = induction; "N/V" = nausea/vomiting; "prodrug" means that the parent compound is metabolized into the active agent; in these cases, inhibition leads to less drug activity.
Strong inhibitors/inducers in bold. Moderate inhibitors/inducers in plain text.

Index

[NOTE] Page numbers followed by *f* indicate figures; *t* indicates a table.

CPSIA information can be obtained
at www.ICGtesting.com
Printed in the USA
LVHW082141150523
747095LV00031B/782

9 781732 952263